"Creative mindfulness practices have been so valuable for taking care of myself as a mental health clinician. The creative process gets me out of my head and allows for different perspectives, problem-solving, and healing of vicarious trauma."

Sara DeWitt, *LPC, CADC I*

"*Healing from Clinical Trauma Using Creative Mindfulness Techniques* is a beautiful, creative, thoughtful, and well written work. It is highly recommended for art therapists who use mindfulness creativity in their work already or are just beginning to develop this practice for themselves."

Kazz Artis, *Art therapist, Artist, Mental health consultant*

"In and out of calendar days and countless therapies; faced with abundant challenges in processing pain, angst & argument around abuse, reframing victimization into victories... Beth Ann's compassionate and supportive guidance through the Creative Mindfulness Technique means of art-making has been transformative. Despite statistically calculating naysayers who'd suggest mental illness outcomes grow progressively more dire with age, I embrace a more hopeful future, in large part to rediscovery, reinvention and renewed purpose founded upon practicing Creative Mindfulness."

Lindsey Grant

Healing from Clinical Trauma Using Creative Mindfulness Techniques

This workbook offers diverse strengths-based tools to incorporate the Creative Mindfulness Technique (CMT) into clinical practice. It provides an essential understanding of the ethical scope of practice, ensuring that clinicians consider the depth of their own training in the implementation of the CMT art directives.

Chapters explore aspects such as attachment and art therapy, multicultural considerations when using art with clients, mindfulness, the eight dimensions of wellness, and the application of CMT techniques with clients affected by PTSD, anxiety, and low self-esteem. The creative activities, mindfulness approaches, and arts-based exercises provided support the healing process of clients in ways that are accessible, practical, and easy to execute. Examples of activities include guided imageries with art-making, art journaling directives, and mixed media prompts. Through these exercises, clients will learn to draw upon their strengths and feel empowered in their daily lives.

People with PTSD/clinical trauma, stress, addiction, and anxiety, and clinicians and mental health practitioners working with them will find this book to be an essential tool.

Corinna M. Costello, Ph.D., LCMHCS, ATR-BC is the director of student support and a core faculty member of clinical mental health at The Family Institute of Northwestern University. Dr. Costello also practices art therapy. She contributed chapters for *The Neuroeducation Toolbox* and *Encyclopedia of Couple and Family Therapy*. She has also written and presented extensively on PTSD, anxiety, resiliency, mindfulness, and art therapy.

Beth Ann Short LCAT, ATR-BC (they/them) is a licensed certified art therapist in Oregon and an adjunct professor in art therapy at Lewis & Clark College in Portland, Oregon and at Heritage University in Toppenish, Washington. Short authored *Creative Wellness: Art Journaling with Mindfulness* in 2016. Short is also a fine artist who has exhibited art both internationally and in publications.

Healing from Clinical Trauma Using Creative Mindfulness Techniques

A Workbook of Tools and Applications

Corinna M. Costello and Beth Ann Short

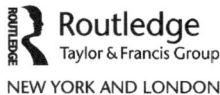

NEW YORK AND LONDON

First published 2022
by Routledge
605 Third Avenue, New York, NY 10158

and by Routledge
2 Park Square, Milton Park, Abingdon, Oxon, OX14 4RN

Routledge is an imprint of the Taylor & Francis Group, an Informa business

© 2022 Taylor & Francis

Library of Congress Cataloging-in-Publication Data
A catalog record for this title has been requested

ISBN: 978-0-367-47829-2 (hbk)
ISBN: 978-0-367-47827-8 (pbk)
ISBN: 978-1-003-03677-7 (ebk)

DOI: 10.4324/9781003036777

Typeset in Times New Roman
by MPS Limited, Dehradun

I dedicate this book to all the clients, supervisees, and students I have worked with over the years. Through their work, I have witnessed vulnerability and bravery. It is truly an honor to have been with each of you on your journey.

A special thank you to my sweet family, Robert, and Brody, for all their continuous support in my many projects and ideas.

And of course thank you to Cori Costello, my dear friend, and writing partner.

Beth Ann Short

Contents

List of Figures   xii
Author's Note   xiv
Preface   xvi

Introduction   1
Introduction 1
  Ethical Use and Scope of Practice 2
  Creativity 3
  Culture and Social Constructivism 4

PART I The Evolution of the Creative Mindfulness Technique   7

1 Art and the Process   9
Attachment and Art Therapy 11
The Expressive Therapies Continuum 13
Art Mediums 14
  Properties of Art Mediums 15
  Art Mediums 16
  What is Mixed Media? 20
Art Directives 20
Multicultural Considerations and the Creative
  Mindfulness Technique 21

2 Mindfulness: Being in the Moment   23
The Unconscious 23
Be Here Now 24
Mindfulness and the Eight Dimensions of Wellness 25
  Emotional Wellness 25
  Social Wellness 26

Spiritual Wellness 28
Intellectual Wellness 29
Environmental Wellness 30
Physical Wellness 31
Occupational Wellness 33
Financial Wellness 33
The Creative Mindfulness Technique 34
The Formal Steps of CMT 34
Alternative Supports Utilized in Mindfulness 35
Neurofeedback 35
Breathwork 36

PART II Applications of the Creative Mindfulness Technique   37

3 Application   39
Post Traumatic Stress Disorder 39
Anxiety 41
Depressive Disorders 42
Grief 43
Low Self-esteem 44
Addiction 45

4 Art Journaling   47
Eight Dimensions of Wellness 48
Gratitude 48
Feeling Check In 49
Self-talk 50
From Worry to Relaxation 51
Ritual 51
Strengths 52
Supporting the 12 Steps 52

5 Guided Imageries   55
Guided Imagery Example 1 Body Scan 55
Guided Imagery Example 2 Variation on an Energy
  Ball 59
Guided Imagery Example 3 Safe Place in Nature 60
Guided Imagery Example 4 Inner Plant 62

6 Tools for Safety   64
Creative Mindfulness Mantra Cards 64

Mandalas 66
Tool Box 68
Safe Space 70

7 Self Reflection   71

This is me, I am... 71
I come from... 72
Beggar Bowl 74
What I Know for Sure 75
Inside/Outside Box 75
I statements 75
Tree 77

8 Externalizing   79

What does _____ look like? 79
Barometer 81
Struggle Container 81
It's OK 83

9 Working with It   85

Planting Seeds 85
My Struggle and My Relationships 85
My Struggle and My Environment 89
Dear _____, 90
Relapse 90
I Want You to Know 92

10 Vicarious Trauma and the Clinician   94

References   104
Index   110

Figures

1.1	Art from the AH:LE Gender Summit	10
1.2	Altered book	17
4.1	Eight dimensions of wellness	48
4.2	Gratitude journal entry	49
4.3	"A Question of Moods"	50
4.4	Self-talk journal entry	51
4.5	Journeys	52
4.6	Self-care rituals journal entry	53
4.7	Strengths	54
5.1	Body outline	56
5.2	Body scan response art	58
5.3	The Center of My Uterus	58
5.4	Energy ball response art 1	60
5.5	Energy ball response art 2	60
5.6	Safe place response art	62
5.7	Inner plant response art	63
6.1	Mindfulness mantra cards	65
6.2	Mandala 1	66
6.3	Mandala 2	68
6.4	Tool box 1	69
6.5	Safe space response art	70
7.1	This is me I am... (1)	72
7.2	I come from...	73
7.3	Beggar bowl	74
7.4	Box	76
7.5	"I" statement game	77
7.6	Trees	78
8.1	What does gender look like?	80
8.2	Barometer	82
8.3	Struggle bottle	83
8.4	Wax resist process	84

9.1	Planting seeds 1	86
9.2	Planting seeds 2	87
9.3	Response art: relationships	88
9.4	Relationships journal entry	88
9.5	Response art: balancing the eight dimensions	89
9.6	Open letter: wax resist	91
9.7	Relapse of emotion	92
10.1	Clinician response art 1: 2020	96
10.2	Clinician response art 1: suicide	97
10.3	Clinician response art: soothing	98
10.4	Clinician response art: transition into professional	99
10.5	Clinician response art: rage	100
10.6	Clinician response art: navigating systems	101
10.7	Clinician response art: tree	102
10.8	Clinician response art: nest	103

Author's Note

Growing up I had never heard of mindfulness, but I had heard of meditation. I remember once while living in Ontario, Canada when I was nine years old coming upon one of my brothers as he sat peacefully in a zen state facing Lake Superior on the rocky shore. I recall feeling as though he was not there even though his body was but in a higher place. I remember quietly leaving, wondering what magic he was experiencing sitting there on the sharp rocks without a care in the world. Much of my childhood was spent at this secluded place in nature infused with sporadic chaos, but also a lot of alone time taking hikes in nature. I realize now that I was lucky to have parents who encouraged creativity. Looking back on that time now I realize my many moments of staring into campfires, looking up at the stars in the sky, witnessing the wildlife around me, or observing the crashing waves on the rocks were a sort of mindfulness. This sounds romantic, but this place I seem to canonize was a safe place and respite from the life we lived. Multiple moves, inconsistent parenting, chaos, loneliness, and trauma underscored a childhood my siblings and I endured telling our stories with bravado to cope and minimize how we felt. My father often said, "Don't look back!" each time we drove away from a home and from friends I had made.

As I grew and we returned to the states I found myself reading books I found in our house that included Henry David Thoreau. I realize now that mindfulness practice was second nature to me as I grew up often utilized as an escape. I find myself now years later a licensed certified art therapist in Oregon with 20+ years of practice behind me having a deeper knowledge of mindfulness, but also a consistent meditation practice that is one of the cornerstones of my own wellness. My work over the years has evolved from working with at-risk youth in foster care and juvenile justice navigating many broken systems, to a more community-based setting in an open studio. It was in this space that I identified the work I had been doing realizing I was doing a form of creative mindfulness not only in my own self-care but also with my clients. In 2016 I wrote and self-published a therapy tool called *Creative Wellness: Art Journaling with Mindfulness.* I had already met Cori Costello and worked with her for a number of years serving on a committee for the Art Therapy Credentials Board (ATCB). She went on to do her dissertation on the Creative Mindfulness Technique. Our work complements each other's and after many discussions around this, here we are. I hope these books serve to support mindfulness in both clients' and clinician's lives.

Beth Ann Short

Preface

The *Creative Mindfulness Techniques for Clinical Trauma Work* and the companion workbook *Healing from Clinical Trauma Using Creative Mindfulness Techniques* (Costello & Short, 2021) explore the interventions of incorporating creativity and mindfulness into clinical mental health work. Through reviewing the evidence, the reader will learn how to consider the safe and effective use of creative and mindful approaches within the clinical setting and understand why these aspects are important to the process of emotional healing within the human species. The interventions presented to support the strengthening of resiliency and wellness considerations in the clinical experience of trauma work.

In reviewing the evidence presented throughout the book *Creative Mindfulness Techniques for Clinical Trauma Work*, the reader will consider why it is important to incorporate some creative and mindful steps into their clinical work. Used in conjunction with the companion treatment planner "Healing from Clinical Trauma Using Creative Mindfulness Techniques" (Costello & Short, 2021), the reader will be offered practical techniques with pragmatic steps to incorporate these interventions safely and effectively in the clinical setting.

In the book *Creative Mindfulness Techniques for Clinical Trauma Work*, we will explore the evidence to support the innate act of the creative process, and the impact of the central nervous system on our human response to survival. Creative Mindfulness techniques will be defined, we will explore the importance of the human experience of creativity from an anthropological look at history and how the *Homo sapiens* species have utilized creativity for communication, expression, and protection. The neurobiological ramification of trauma on the body and brain will be discussed and we will examine how humans respond and adapt to stress and its impact over long periods of time.

Approaches to finding balance or *allostasis* within the central nervous system will be explored including changing stress-inducing behaviors through neuroplasticity, breathwork, and mindfulness. Further evidence will examine the importance of mindful approaches and how other researchers have viewed these mindful activities throughout history. We will discuss how other authors have viewed and incorporated creativity and mindfulness techniques into their clinical work. Next, the considerations for building resiliency and the impact this construct may have on the individual dealing with trauma, from a neurophysiological perspective. Finally, the book will provide case examples to demonstrate the utilization of the Creative Mindfulness Techniques. These examples include Creative Mindfulness Techniques for supervision purposes, self-awareness and cultural considerations, the integration of mindfulness, the traumatized client experience, journaling for self-reflection, and poetry for the professional development of a counselor.

The companion workbook *Healing from Clinical Trauma Using Creative Mindfulness Techniques* (Costello & Short, 2021) will provide ethical, cultural, social constructivism considerations for creativity and mindful approaches in clinical trauma work and potentially comorbid issues related to trauma. This workbook will offer strength-based techniques and healing approaches while guiding the experience through creativity and mindfulness techniques. It will provide mental health clinicians opportunities to utilize various techniques, in conjunction with treatment, or as a companion homework approach.

The workbook explores the incorporation of creativity and mindfulness techniques through a process-driven approach. Also examined, is the attachment style presented in psychodynamic theory and art therapy, as well as the transitional object consideration of clinical focus. Next, the book explores the utilization of the art directive and concern for the material or media choice within the clinical experience. The processing of the experience of creative moments as well as the product created from the session will be discussed.

Mindfulness and being in the moment are examined from an unconscious perspective and the eight dimensions of wellness, including breath work, and neurofeedback. The eight dimensions of wellness are emotions, social relationships, spirituality, intellectual wellness, the environment, the physical wellness of the body, occupation, and finances.

The workbook outlines and describes the *Creative Mindfulness Technique and* steps for effectiveness, as well as provide direct examples of guided imagery and directives. Also provided in this workbook are steps for assisting clients impacted with self-esteem issues and art directives that increase self-confidence goals. The workbook will further explore various pragmatic examples of clinical techniques for use with clients dealing with various other mental health concerns and diagnoses including anxiety, unipolar and bipolar disorder, post-traumatic stress disorder (PTSD), grief and loss, and addiction concerns.

Introduction

Introduction

Mindfulness has become a popular term in lifestyle, health, and wellness over the past decade. Buddhist in origination, the term came from the word "sati" in Pali, an ancient language of India and means "awareness." Jon Kabat-Zinn, influential for bringing mindfulness to the west, developed his Mindfulness-Based Stress Reduction (MBSR) program, where an individual intentionally pays attention to purpose, without judgment (1990, 1994). This movement stimulated a surge of mindfulness practices in the field of counseling. The Creative Mindfulness Technique (CMT) developed by Dr. Corinna Costello, has evolved through the blending of mindfulness techniques with clinical art therapy.

This CMT treatment planner partner to Costello's book, *Creative Mindfulness Techniques for Clinical Trauma Work,* provides interactive mindfulness tools blended with art therapy and provides a deeper understanding of the CMT approach (Costello, 2021). The process utilizes grounding techniques, mindfulness meditations, art therapy directives, and verbal processes as a conduit in the therapeutic process. "The goal with this interactive method is to increase psychological health and develop self-actualization skills for the clinical mental health client" (Costello, 2015). The objectives of this book partnered with *Creative Mindfulness Techniques for Clinical Trauma Work*, are to provide an engaging tool that is approachable and ethical for mental health professionals in their practice with traumatized clients as well as in their own self-care. The book is divided into 2 parts, Part I provides an overview of influences and the development of CMT. Chapter 1 provides information about art, art mediums, and the process. Chapter 2 furnishes a more detailed exploration of mindfulness practices, the eight dimensions of wellness, and a delineation of the Creative Mindfulness Technique. Part II explores specific trauma-based diagnoses and conflicts, describing how art therapy and meditation have been beneficial in the treatment and then expands upon art directives that may be used with the CMT. Chapter 10 closes the book with a variety of art created by clinicians for their own

DOI: 10.4324/9781003036777-101

self-care in response to vicarious trauma experienced through their work or outside influences.

Ethical Use and Scope of Practice

The Art Therapy Credentials Board (ATCB) is the national board that art therapists are credentialed through in the United States. The ATCB ethics state, "Art therapists are encouraged, whenever possible, to promote public understanding of the principles and the profession of art therapy through presentations to general audiences, mental health professionals, and students. In making such presentations, art therapists shall accurately convey to the audience members or students the expected competence and qualifications that will result from the presentations, as well as, the differences between the presentation and formal studies in art therapy" (Art Therapy Credentials Board, N. D., Code 1.5.8). Any clinicians' first priority is to protect the public. Art therapists are trained not only to protect the public but also to educate. There is a constant reminder throughout the art therapy community to act with caution when sharing the details of the practice with providers who do not have specialized art therapy degrees. The American Art Therapy Association (AATA) cautions credentialed art therapists in its ethics, "When providing training and/or supervision to non-art therapists, art therapists take precautions to ensure that trainees understand the nature, objectives, expectations, limitations and resulting qualifications of the supervision and/or training as distinct from formal studies in art therapy" (American Art Therapy Association, N. D.).

It is vital that those without art therapy training work with extreme caution in how art is incorporated into practice with clients. While art therapists do not own art, they do provide clients a different perspective that considers the properties of media, which can invoke a wide variety of reactions from clients. For those curious about art therapy, additional training should be required. All licensed mental health professionals have the duty to attain continuing education credits annually to continue to grow and evolve into seasoned professionals throughout their careers. These continuing education classes/training present clinicians outside of the field the opportunities to follow interests that are symbiotic with their own professional aesthetic. One's professional aesthetic refers to the integration of clinical theories that may inform one's approach in working with their clients. This aesthetic may also be seen as the way in which they create a safe place for their clients.

Additionally one might consider looking into becoming a Registered Art Therapist (ATR), as one does not have to have a master's in art therapy as long as they have fulfilled the educational and supervisory requirements established by the ATCB. Details can be found on the ATCB website. When choosing to incorporate art into the counseling practice the clinician should strongly consider what outcomes to goals they anticipate achieving. Choice of materials without consideration into the properties of media may result in outcomes not anticipated. Springham outlines a case where a practitioner who was not a trained art therapist utilized art with a client that then resulted in a psychotic event (2008). The client who engaged in the process believed the clinician to be a trusted advocate as they were already in a fragile state with limits in reality testing and had whole-heartedly committed to the work looking for support during a difficult time. A legal case followed due to the practitioner's lack of expertise in assessing the client's mental state and taking into consideration how the art directive utilized might impact them (Springham, 2008). It is vital to re-member that the power dynamic in the therapeutic relationship, clients trust that professionals are working within their scope of practice and are committed to doing no harm.

Creativity

Art therapy can be sought out for many reasons. A common mis-conception about the approach is that it is only for children. Art therapy is for anyone. An art therapist's training encompasses master's level clinical counseling skills plus a thorough understanding of the complex properties of art materials and how to use them. Work with clients is personalized to their needs. Often many who come to an art therapist are in search of an alternative to traditional counseling. There is no art ex-perience necessary. Clients may be initially anxious about creating art. In early assessment, the clinician works to get a solid understanding of the client's strengths and struggles, which significantly impact the choice of art medium and directives to be used in treatment. In sessions, art therapists provide demonstrations of art mediums for their clients before the client engages in art-making. A significant undercurrent in art therapy is encouraging the process and that creativity is a choice. The clinician must be able to create and provide a space for the therapeutic relationship to grow and thrive, fostering conditions where creative risks may be taken. A more detailed exploration on this and how art therapy can be a conduit in working through broken childhood attachments to come in Chapter 1.

Humans use creativity every day without acknowledging it. It may surface in ways that are not art-based, but creativity is essential in problem-solving. Creativity is not limited to being employed by humans solely as an art-based experience but is initiated in all forms of problem-solving in daily life. In the counseling arena art therapists and clients both use creativity in developing and maintaining the therapeutic relationship, creating goals in treatment, and implementing directives or tools that may transmute into a sustainable practice in daily life. When we are creative we are birthing ideas from our imagination into our reality. The creative process provides opportunities to explore, problem solves, and perhaps make connections while solving problems. Shore explores the role of the art therapist not only as a trained professional supporting the creative process but also taking into consideration creativity and its impact on the brain fostering the integration of both brain hemispheres (2014). "Such integrative approaches are necessary for attempting repair of early relational trauma" (Shore, 2014, p. 94). The process Shore describes is another type of creativity. Art therapists utilize their clinical training as well as their expertise with art media to guide clients through the process. Hinz associates creative work as an opportunity to increase an individual's "inclusion in the dominant culture, promote posttraumatic growth, (and) enhance self-esteem" (2017). Hinz goes on to explore the concept of creativity as a "human right and force for positive change" (2017). The emphasis in her writing indicates the opportunity for inclusion and its personification by the art therapists who must provide a safe space where clients have the right to express concerns through the art process. In art therapy, there is more to the experience than creating an art product. The clinicians' creativity must also be active as they engage and adapt to their client's needs.

All clinicians must embrace the unexpected when working with clients being consistently flexible, in art therapy, this includes fostering the creative process as it occurs and evolves with an understanding that the product may not exude novelty to them, but will have meaning on some level for the client. Creativity, when embraced, is manifested by choice and is not solely linked to an artistic expression but may be linked to any action in that creativity actively promotes change to any plan, action, or product transforming the existing experience (Csikszentmihalyi, 1996; Short, 2016).

Culture and Social Constructivism

The therapeutic stage also provides space for clients to shine a light on their unique stories and backgrounds and how they may play into their need for support. Inclusion is also a major factor in creating a safe incorporating astute consideration supporting each client's unique intersections when choosing the optimum art medium and directives. Art therapists reference the Expressive Therapies Continuum (Chapter 1) to consider the appropriateness of media and art directive, although this continuum is not equipped to explore how creativity is impacted by cultural influences. The therapeutic choices clinicians make must come from a professional open to continuous learning and self-reflection. A therapist's inherent intersections and personal narrative are unwittingly and unconsciously present in the therapeutic space. A therapist must frequently examine and explore their professional identity to understand the impact they have, as they are a culmination of their intentions behind becoming a clinician as well as their own narrative and life intersections.

Shore surmised that both "personal and social/cultural/political factors underlie human strengths and pathologies" (2006, p. 177). A clinician's personal growth and limitations may affect clients, as well as the state of the world and systems that hold power over the Earth's inhabitants (Shore, 2006).

Karcher affirms the work of a clinician including validation in a society where clients have experienced oppression and trauma (2017). In the work of externalizing potentially oppressive messages, the clinician provides a space for clients to build a "sense of agency and power" (Karcher, 2017). It is vital for clinicians to examine their own privilege, power, and intersections throughout their life and career. A clinician's experience of the norm is likely to differ from the client's personal experience and may have included access to opportunities nonexistent to clients. Each individual's experience of financial/ socioeconomic status; race; sexual orientation; gender expression; citizenship; religion; physical, social, emotional, or cognitive challenges; or age may strongly differ creating a power hierarchy that must be considered to avoid contamination in the therapeutic alliance (Karcher, 2017; Ter Maat, 2011). Comprehending, valuing, and recognizing the many intersections an in-dividual carries with them provides heightened insights including "a sig-nificant bidirectional relationship with biological, characterological, familial, and societal systems" (Berg-Cross et al., 2001, p. 849).

Multicultural competence encompasses a combination of cultural aware-ness, knowledge, and skills (Sue et al., 1982; Sue & Sue, 2008; Ter Maat, 2011). To offer multicultural competent support services clinicians should examine each of these in detail. Cultural self-awareness is only the beginning to overall cultural awareness. Clinicians must examine their own assumptions about human behavior and nature as well as explore foundational values, beliefs, and attitudes towards their culture and the cultural experiences that shaped them (Sue & Sue, 2008; Ter Maat, 2011). Expanding cultural knowledge should also be an ongoing practice in the clinician's development to ensure they are providing an engaging multicultural safe space. Clinicians must take the initiative to explore and understand the cultural norms, atti-tudes, and world views of all clients. This contributes to the foundation of the therapeutic alliance and recognizes and honors these views with validation. Lastly, through this ongoing self-study cultural skills gained will provide outlets to therapeutic techniques, tasks, and tools to use in clinical work (Ter Maat, 2011). Art therapists have the training to adapt art directives perso-nalizing them to meet each client's needs and whose backgrounds may differ from the art therapist's. Cultural factors of clients may affect individual and family treatment planning and outcomes (McGoldrick & Hardy, 2008). These may include language spoken at home, socioeconomic status, level of education, practiced method of processing or not processing emotionally charged materials, political beliefs, and religious practices. Additional cultu-rally sensitive skills can be attained by attending continuing educational training after graduation throughout career, participating in supervision and consultation, and engaging in deliberate research to synthesize concepts of the life experience of others.

A multicultural sensitive practice provides opportunities for ongoing growth seeing the differences from a psychological perspective, but even deeper from social and cultural points of view (Talwar, 2010). A socially active clinician should embody an understanding of the impacts of social, cultural, and political pressures and how they impact each client personally. One can experience many types of intersections occurring in both macro and micro social structures that provide insights into the many social locations and experiences that do not conform to middle-class stereotypes. The acknowledgment of these social locations provides opportunities for individuals to be seen and acknowledged for who they truly are. Actively working to deepen an understanding of the lives and experiences of marginalized humans through a thorough examination of influences may better impact future access to opportunities and services (Thornton-Dill & Zambrana, 2009). Inequalities that may stem from race, ethnicity, class, gender, and religion historically have impacted access providing those with privileged benefits honoring exclusivity and group membership.

Each clinician must address underlying biases in their own intersections when working to meet clients where they are using "intersectional scholarship" (Thornton-Dill & Zambrana, 2009, p. 2). In this ever-growing process, each person must embrace a social justice mission that seeks to reinvent their self-prescribed values and ideas relating to humankind and relationships integrating the wide variety of experiences lived by all in society at large. In clinical work and beyond clinicians must consider their role in society and how they participate and advocate for those they work with. Cultural competency in clinical practice includes sensitivity in choosing art media and directives and not imposing extreme or stereotypical themes of culture and the creative process (Kapitan, 2015; Talwar, 2015). Additionally, what may be perceived as creative in one culture may not be in another. In some cultures, the expression of creativity is seen as a novelty and not as valued as it is not aligned with usefulness or prosperity (Kwan et al., 2018).

Ultimately, clinicians must have a deep awareness of their own power and privilege that may extend outside of the therapeutic relationship. Clinicians are responsible to deeply assess their own truths and how those truths may impact the therapeutic bond (Karcher, 2017). A deep ongoing self-reflective practice around privilege, race and the many intersections must be challenged and exercised throughout the career of a clinician to ensure one is meeting clients in place with unequivocal tolerance and respect at all times.

Part I

The Evolution of the Creative Mindfulness Technique

1   Art and the Process

What interests us about other people's art? It is common to consider the artist's motivations when looking at a piece of art. Museums and galleries worldwide exhibit art for the public to view and contemplate. How is their art different from the art created in an art therapy session? Some isn't, but some is and comes from a product driven approach utilizing the formal elements of art looking to create balance and symmetry in an art form. In art school students attend critiques where art is thoroughly examined by the instructor and peers in the class. Critiques are learning opportunities for students exploring the art product in relation to media technique, however the process is not always deeply considered. In art therapy the product may be experienced like an iceberg, what lies beneath represents a vast array of experiences, truths, feelings, thoughts, and intentions. The process is not limited to art therapy in the creation a piece of art. For instance, consider artists like Egon Shiele or Frida Kahlo. They were artists who created pieces of art in response to their life experiences and self-concept. Humans are still fascinated by their work. Many artists do channel the process having no formal training, they have been labeled *outsider artists* (Cardinal, 1972). The term comes from writer and historian Roger Cardinal who described an *outsider artist* as one who has no formal training and lives outside of the confines of the art world (Cardinal, 1972). While human creativity continues to evolve outside of traditional art, some in the art world continue to look the other way from outsider art not valuing the process that is often an undercurrent in art-making. Art therapy embraces the process.

Typically art made in an art therapy session is not put on display, and is considered confidential in content, as important as the client's words in session. In open studios the lines of confidentiality become less rigid, dependent on the agreement between the client and art therapist. Releases must be signed for art to be hung for display or used in educational situations. Open studio projects like the Artist/Humankind: Location/ Earth (AH:LE) provide platforms for stories to reach others feeling alone and marginalized. This project aims to provide anyone "the opportunity to share their own life experiences using a creative outlet and find community in the process" (Short, n. d.). The goals of the project inclusive to

DOI: 10.4324/9781003036777-1

anyone who comes into contact to view the art as well as the participants (Short, n. d.):

- Participants will experience increased ability to use creativity in self-care, as well as in problem solving while gaining insight into past, present and future life choices through this process.
- Participants will explore self-perception and personal role identity formation exploring and engaging with others in the core group finding normalcy in their experience relating to the role of the session, while translating their own experience in their unique art voice.
- Participants will examine the concept of roles in life that guide our behaviors, rights and obligations through the social experience in social status, social community and expectations of others.

Participants were not required to have any experience using art materials. The ongoing project currently has completed three versions of the project including the Caregiver Summit, the Gender Summit (Figure 1.1),

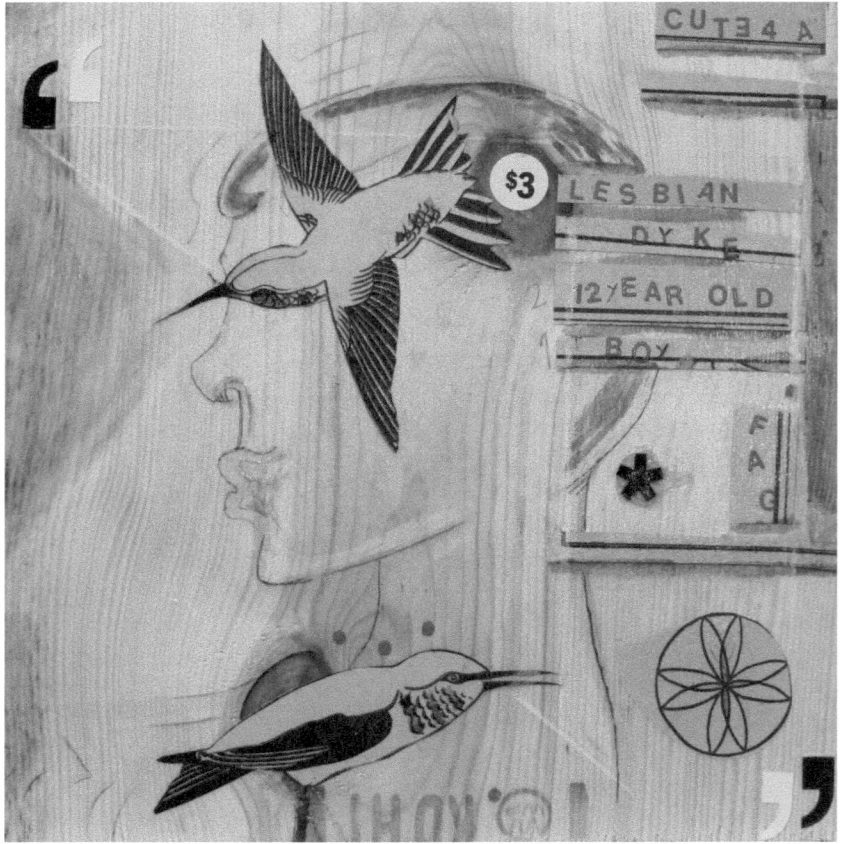

Figure 1.1 Art from the AH:LE Gender Summit.

and the Survivor Summit. Each session consists of a period of group art-making over a period of time and then an exhibition. The Gender Summit went on to travel to multiple locations providing educational talks about the experience including a panel discussion of select participants at one conference. In each of the sessions project participants were not individual therapy clients, signing releases prior to starting the process. All art pieces remained the artists' property once the session ended.

Art provides a limitless container for humankind to communicate about needs, desires, events and experiences. Humans have been creating art for over 40,000 years. What motivates the creation or the urge to observe art? Could it be as simple as finding a familiar thought, feeling, intention, or experience? To not be alone in this life? Art therapy provides opportunities for clients to use the process as an additional voice in treatment. Traditional counseling does not work for everyone. Not all clients are able or open to sitting and talking. Art therapy becomes an engaging vehicle or *transitional object* in the therapeutic process (Robbins, 1998). The art process and exploring materials has been fundamental for some clients to challenge existing patterns (Pénzes et al., 2014). Arthur Robbins implicates object relations art therapy as his version of art therapy pulling from psycho-analytic theory whereas the art process becomes the object where a person's "libidinal energy is invested" (p. 131). Robbins compares the art therapy process to that of a transitional object to a child. As a child emotes, plays, imagines, practices, socializes, and projects onto that transitional object, the object in turn is an accepting non-judgmental vessel. The art therapy process is also that, a safe malleable container, or object of attachment. The process provides room for clients to explore struggles around separation, individuation, dependence, independence, and intimacy thus providing opportunities to repair developmental deficiencies from early childhood relationships (Robbins, 2016). "Art can contain, organize, and mirror internal object relations and the interplay between therapist, client, and the art product" (Robbins, 2012, p. 70).

Attachment and Art Therapy

Ruptured childhood attachments appear to be underlying in many diagnoses, especially those that are trauma based. Secure attachment not only allows an infant the ability to begin to individually regulate their emotions, but it also is vital in the development of the brain (Malchiodi, 2012a). A child with secure attachment is more resilient in facing adversity. Resilience has been defined as an individual's ability to understand, anticipate, and then cope with a traumatic event, which may be by threat or stress (Agaibi & Wilson, 2005). Attachment can be connected to both psychological and physiological experiences. Many sensory memories stored in the limbic system may be accessed through art therapy and can be crucial in working through struggles. The art therapy process has been perceived to contribute successful completion of treatment goals. The process is known to reduce anxiety around treatment as well as expedite the formation of the therapeutic relationship. Art therapy has also been proven to increase memory recovery and details surrounding experiences (Malchiodi, 2012a).

Siegel outlined four components of attachment that individuals who have secure attachment experience, they are being seen, feeling safe, receiving soothing, and feeling secure (Siegel, 2010). Secure attachment is one of four types of attachment that individuals experience; the others are avoidant, ambivalent, and disorganized attachment (Siegel, 2010). Some individuals may be likely to experience a combination of these considering there may be multiple caregivers in their childhood. Caregivers may include biological parents, but may also include stepparents, partners of parents, grandparents, aunts, uncles, older siblings, and cousins. Individuals who experience secure attachment have felt consistently secure, seen and soothed in their needs and experience of life as they develop from infancy. Seigel notes that a child who experiences avoidant attachment has a caregiver who is indifferent to them and does not respond to their needs (Siegel, 2010). In ambivalent attachment, parents are inconsistent sometimes engaged and available while other times tuned out (Siegel, 2010). Disorganized attachment seems to add to an individual's trauma narrative more than the others due to the caregiver's extreme lack of attunement creating a frightening environment often filled with chaos that develops into degraded representations that can elicit strong emotional reactions perpetuating a vehement cycle involving both the body and the mind (Siegel, 2010; van der Kolk, 2014). Attachment work in mental health treatment can provide individuals who have experienced one or more of the insecure forms of attachment an opportunity to make sense of both their inner and external worlds.

Art therapy treatment can provide an opportunity to address these broken attachments. As formerly mentioned engaging the process is akin to the concept of a transitional object. The art therapist provides materials in a safe space and becomes a part of the play of recreating opportunities to address these broken attachments. When epistemic experiences happen consistently there is more success in attachment work. Springham & Huet propose an alignment with art therapy and the bio-psychosocial model noting the creation and development of art pieces as *second-order representations* (2018). These works transform into a mechanism that impacts the attachment system, however, the therapist must embrace their role as an attachment provider. As previously mentioned, an art therapist has the specialized training, which supports the client's trust in the process. Providing a safe space creates an environment where clients feel more readily able to trust and more prepared to make disclosures in relation to the process. The trained art therapist knows the importance of being concise in comments focusing more on the client's responses to the process and artwork (Springham & Huet, 2018).

Art therapists utilize art directives in their work with clients. An art therapy directive is a thematic prompt and chosen specifically for each client, as each client has unique intersections that makeup who they are. This treatment planner includes examples of directives that will require sensitive consideration prior to implementation. Art therapy is not a formula. While there are many formal methods of assessment, each individual brings with them their experiences, strengths, and struggles. Art therapy formal training, supervision, and consultation provide a structure for art therapist's evolving professional identities fostering growth resulting in a seasoned professional with an intricate understanding of clinical art therapy and its application to each unique individual they encounter. Through the use of art directives clients take creative risks within the safe structure of the session while making art and also discussing the process. It should be stressed that art directives may impact individuals differently. The process includes multiple factors like the client's overall effect, how they may be emoting throughout the session from beginning to end. It includes the client's behavior, which includes how they interact with media. The process involves the client's cognitive functioning, including problem-solving in using media or in immediate conversation. Additionally, the process includes social or familial undertones that may surface throughout the session in conversation or in the art. To be clear, art therapists do not analyze their client's art. They talk with their clients and ask clarifying questions to support the process.

The process is not a scripted curriculum for use in a similar fashion with each client. This therapeutic process becomes conformable and accommodating to each client's needs.

Annette Shore considers the art therapy process as one that involves tolerance providing the client an honored witness in the process that brings about "strengthening and renewing one's sense of meaning" (2006, p. 189). The creative risks clients take in the process, in turn, serve as stepping stones of choice that contribute to building resiliency. This practice impacts the client to be more readily able to confront and address trauma or other struggles impacting daily functioning. Some art directives may be more approachable earlier in treatment, while others may be better utilized after the therapeutic alliance is established.

The Expressive Therapies Continuum

The Expressive Therapies Continuum (ETC), developed by Sandra Kagin and Vija Lusebrink, is an assessment tool used in art therapy treatment that is focused on an individual's creative functioning (Lusebrink, 1990, 2010; Hinz, 2020). This tool, in theory, is based on human development and information processing and focuses on conceptualizing an individual's creative functioning. Snir and Regev (2013) describes the ETC as a "systemic approach to understand the relationship between client and materials" (p. 94). It is based on exploring the artist's purpose for creating a piece, the medium chosen, the synergy of the artist's approach to the chosen medium, and the narrative or imagery within the art product (Malchiodi, 2012b).

An art therapist utilizes the ETC to determine which mediums and art directives are appropriate for each client and also provides clinicians with information about how a client's brain processes imagery within their sensory-motor development, cognition, and psychosocial behavior (Lusebrink, 1990, 2010; Malchiodi 2012b; Hinz, 2020). The ETC is divided into levels including (1) the kinesthetic/sensory level, (2) the perceptual/affective level, (3) the cognitive/symbolic level, and the (4) creative level (Lusebrink, 1990, 2010). The continuum is read from left to right and from the bottom upwards and flows in a manner that takes into consideration simple information processing and image creation to progressively more complex thought processes and problem-solving with the art medium (Lusebrink, 1990, 2010; Malchiodi, 2012b; Hines, 2020). As a client engages in the art process they are assessed in the manner in which they register on each section. Each line can be seen as a range, the centerline exemplifying balance between the descriptors. An individual may lean more into one side or experience balance. There is not one correct experience sought after in the measurement, in fact, any experience is legitimate and informs the clinician where each individual lies afterward the clinician is then able to discern what mediums and directives may be the most appropriate for an individual (Lusebrink, 1990, 2010; Malchiodi 2012b; Hines, 2020). Lusebrink named the top level of the continuum the Creative level seeing it as the integration of all the levels, each subsequent level equally incorporated (1990).

Art Mediums

In an art therapy session, there are many factors that should be considered. Offices should have proper ventilation, lighting, and access to water. The clinician should also have proper storage, as the art clients create is another form of their words and should be stored in a locked and safe setting. Incorporating art materials also brings with it knowledge of any hazards or toxicity of art materials. Some pigments should not get on the skin and clinicians must put forth an effort to protect their clients and follow any safety requirements of state and federal agencies that might apply to their practice/business. The choice of media for each client is instrumental in the therapeutic process. Prior to entering an art therapy graduate program, candidates must have a large concentration in both fine art and psychology. This provides students with a firm foundation when learning how art therapy can be applied to various clinical theories and the appropriate populations. An art therapist has a deep understanding of the spectrum of art mediums and while one is not better than the other, one may be better than the other when considering each client's strengths and struggles. There are a wide variety of materials to work within the expressive arts. Each medium has properties that can impact a person and can be categorized in a variety of ways. These properties can have a diverse range of reactions depending on the person (Hinz, 2015). A client's perception of an art material may also impact their engagement, for some messiness interferes with the process (Snir & Regev, 2013). A deep understanding of art mediums and their use in an art therapy practice comes with training and experience. With this knowledge comes an understanding of when it is appropriate to pause an activity and re-engage with a different media, or gently support the client through the struggle that may be timely in treatment providing the space for a risk they may be ready to take in building on resilience.

A client who may be feeling depressed and anxious may better benefit from a media that is more controllable like collage than a media they are unable to control like chalk pastels. Part of the training of an art therapist is being able to read the client and know when to present media that may be out of a client's comfort zone to provide a safe opportunity to work with this tension. Knowing if and when to do this comes with training and experience.

Properties of Art Mediums

Controllable vs. fluid: Controllable mediums provide the artist with the opportunity to change their art as they go. Drawing with a pencil and having an eraser to make corrections provides opportunities for gains in confidence for the right client, the wrong client may feel restrained. Fluid media like ink can also have a varied range of reactions. One may experience feelings of frustration if the medium flows in areas that the artist does not want it (e.g. like ink or watercolor on wet paper) whereas for some clients the honoring the spontaneity may result in feelings of empowerment.

Indelible vs. easy to change: Creating an art piece with metal embossing takes patience and focus. Etching a design into the tin creates an enduring image. When a client works in collage the process may be layered with images and words that can be covered up or taken away making the piece forgiving and flexible.

Simple vs. complex: Using tape or staples to add to an art project provides instant gratification. Weaving fiber is a much more complex task requiring the artist to focus on the process of repeatedly layering the fiber to create a larger piece of fabric. Media with simple properties may also be more fitting for clients who have any struggles with fine motor skills.

Structured vs. unstructured: Some art processes involve steps, for instance in printmaking an artist must first come up with a sketch, before transferring the image to the block it will be carved into and then printed from. Mixed media collage is more unstructured and involves layering collage images, drawing, and painting materials. It can also include a wide variety of other media (e.g. glitter, fabric, stickers) depending on the artist's desire.

Soft vs. saturated color: Different mediums produce different intensities of color. The color can impact the mood and overall tone of an art piece. Colored pencils appear lighter in tone on the paper requiring the artists to layer if they want to build up to richer colors, unlike markers that saturate surfaces with bright hues.

Linework vs. swaths of color: Some design markers have assorted tip sizes and archival inks that provide the artist with the ability to create fine lines while a medium like watercolor or chalk pastels provides rich color quickly and in large areas as desired.

Small vs. large motor activity: Sewing materials, pencil, or fine tip design markers are all examples of media that might be involved smaller and tighter movements. Standing up and working at an easel painting or using charcoal would involve larger more gestural movements actions not all clients may not be physically able to perform.

Art Mediums

Art mediums can range from traditional mediums found in art supply stores to found objects and mixed media. Early in treatment, it is best, to begin with, more controllable materials. As treatment progresses, mediums used may evolve as is appropriate in client progress, strengths, and struggles. As already stated different art materials can evoke a wide range of feelings and/or memories in clients, some positive and others difficult (Snir, 2013). The way in which a client engages with materials expresses much about the client including self-worth, independence, rigidity, coping mechanisms, and emotional expression (Pénzes et al., 2014). This section outlines a wide variety of art mediums and art projects but is not likely to be complete. Not all are art therapy directives, however art therapists are creative and always coming up with innovative ways to address treatment needs specific to a client's goals.

Books: Bookmaking provides a containable space to explore the multidimensional minutia of a client's narrative. These books may also serve as art journals. Clients may engage in bookmaking or they may repurpose an existing book creating an *altered book*. Second-hand stores are an excellent place to retrieve them, children's board books are extremely durable and some may have details (e.g. window cutouts, sensory samples) that can be incorporated into the client's process. Children's books often have fewer pages providing a more limited amount of space to address treatment goals topics. Figure 1.2 illustrates a children's book transformed   into   an   emotion-laden   self-narrative.   Handmade

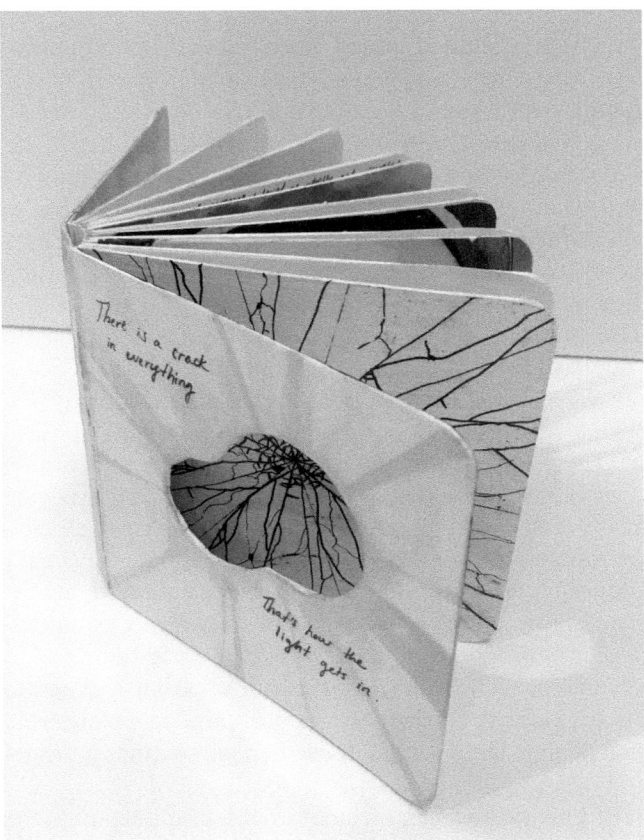

Figure 1.2 Altered book.

bookmaking can vary from extremely sophisticated book-making tech-niques to easy and approachable variations.

Bowls and other vessels: Can often be found at second-hand stores and provide a durable container utilized in treatment to contain struggles or conflicts (see Part II).

Boxes: Boxes can vary from plain cardboard or fancy gift boxes to wooden cigar boxes to more elaborate treasure chest styles. These can often be found at second-hand stores or smoke shops. Boxes may be used to create environments or be symbols for the self.

Clay: Clay provides a wide variety from traditional clay to air-dry options, plasticine, or homemade salt dough. Clay may be used to hand-build or throw on a wheel. Clay has been known to evoke a wide variety of sensory, emotional, and psychological responses in clients and should be implemented into treatment with care.

Collage: Epherma (e.g. collected paper memorabilia), photographs (original or copies), magazines, newspaper, junk mail, colored paper, tissue paper, wrapping paper, maps, children's books. This list goes on and on. Collage is a highly controllable art medium. It is quickly satisfying in that clients may cut out images and words that resonate with them leaving behind what does not. The process can be very inviting to those with little art experience. Many art therapists have pre-cut images prepared for clients to maximize therapy time and avoid clients getting lost looking through magazines.

Digital media: Drawing or painting on a tablet can provide options to clients who might not have access to the materials but have the desire. Some hospital settings have large touch screen options they can wheel directly into patient rooms providing accessible options that include those with a limited range of movement. These devices have programs with movement detection and reaction that sense limited range (e.g. someone in a wheelchair). Digital media may also incorporate storytelling with video, although not all clinicians may have the training or experience necessary to support the client's process and should only be incorporated into treatment with proper training. Uncompleted projects due to the clinician's negligence could adversely impede the client's progress and sense of empowerment.

Doll and puppet making: This ancient art form creating a creature (humanoid or not) provides the maker the opportunity to incorporate specific and personal details. Dolls and puppets then may be incorporated into play therapy.

Drawing materials: This vast list can include pencils, graphite, markers, oil pastels, chalk pastels, design markers, pen, and ink to start. Drawing materials come in their own spectrum from controllable to uncontrollable. A client with sensory struggles may experience an extreme reaction to a messy medium like chalk pastels vs. pencil.

Fiber: Sewing materials, knitting/crochet, fabric collage. Consideration and care for those who may have struggles with fine motor skills. Adaptations to large plastic needles and looser thread counts in the fabric have been an excellent substitute promoting the safe use of a material that may have been off-limits in the past. Fiber materials usually require focus and attention. Some clients may find experience relaxing and self-soothing, while others may struggle with the deep concentration required.

Found objects: This is just what it sounds like. Found objects may be natural or man-made. Some clients may wish to bring items in to incorporate into their projects (e.g. a repurposed broken handheld mirror decorated with positive messages and images to enhance self-worth).

Glass: Glasswork can be fused using a kiln. Glasswork could also be used in the traditional stained glass technique, blown, or used in mosaic.

This media requires experienced supervision and support and is not a typical art medium provided in art therapy sessions.

Masks and body casting: The most popular choice for materials used in art therapy tends to be pre-plastered gauze strips available in arts and craft stores. Plastic face molds are available for those who struggle with the idea of the wet material on their own face. Masks may or may not be humanoid. Some may have an adverse reaction to the sensation of the material on their hands but could wear gloves. Often both the inside and the outside of masks are decorated personifying self-image (e.g. outside: what you should the world; inside: private self). Paint and mixed media are most often utilized in finishing a mask.

Metal embossing: An accessible version of art therapy would be using tin sheets wrapped around a foam core. This is a multistep process involving drawing, tooling and finally, ink is rubbed into the crevices to finish the process. Tools to emboss are required as well as a great deal of focus when transferring a drawing to the metal. The more detail the more elaborate the piece. This medium is definitely not for everyone and less common in art therapy. The process can be seen as tedious, especially for those who may have a hard time focusing.

Painting materials: Paints come in a wide variety. Traditionally, art therapists seem to gravitate towards acrylic and watercolor because of the speed of drying. Additionally, there are many options for water-soluble drawing materials to be combined with acrylic and watercolor paint. Oil paint is less popular in art therapy. Oil paints require more support considering the length of time they take to dry, the need for ventilation, and the potential for exposure to harmful toxins. Some newer versions of water-miscible oil paint can be thinned and cleaned up with water.

Performance art: There is a wide variety of performance art in the expressive arts therapies which may include theatre, music, dance, storytelling, opera, musical theatre, magic, mime, puppetry, improv, comedy, and circus arts. Some artists also engage in performance art in their art expression.

Photography: Traditional photography with a film camera might still include using a dark room when an artist has the option, although this is very rare in art therapy. Digital photography has become an accessible option for many, some using a smartphone rather than a camera. Many individuals display their photos on social media to express who they are or who they want to be. In art therapy, social media should be approached with thoughtful consideration, as it may contribute to struggles clients have (e.g. addiction, social anxiety, low self-esteem). Social media has also provided a platform for bullying.

Printmaking: This art process takes multiple steps first creating a drawing, then carving it onto a surface (e.g. linoleum, wood, Styrofoam). Once the details have been added the surface is covered with ink and then printed onto paper. Fine arts generally create a limited series of prints increasing the value of the work. Printmaking is another of the mediums more rarely used in art therapy.

Sculpture: Sculpture is an art that is three-dimensional. A wide variety of media may be utilized (natural or man-made). Some sculpture involves the craving of an object from a larger piece (e.g. stone or wood) while sculpt adding pieces together. In art therapy, accessible options may include found objects and hot glue.

What is Mixed Media?

Mixed media is an assortment of art materials used in combination. It is important to remember the different properties of art mediums when combining them (e.g. oil based vs. water-soluble). It is vital to have an understanding of what potential reactions may occur in combinations in order to support clients using mixed media in their work. Many mixed media techniques are included in Part II. It is consequential to have watercolor or mixed media paper for clients when layering media. Standard drawing paper is great for drawing materials but may wear thin with layering and too much moisture. This could impact the client's process resulting in regression. Mixed media materials usually include the following:

- Drawing Materials
- Painting materials
- Adhesives: glue stick, white glue, decoupage medium, masking tape, clear tape, washi tape
- Glitter
- Stencils
- Collage materials
- Envelopes
- Sewing materials
- A hairdryer to dry work in between layers

When working with mixed media in an art journal it is a good idea to insert larger sheets of paper to protect the pages on either side of the section being worked on. This will avoid media bleed into other pages as well as avoiding pages getting stuck together.

Art Directives

Part II of this treatment planner is comprised of the CMT art directives that incorporate mindfulness on some level. Each will include the rationale for utilizing the directive and some basic instructions, which will be incorporated into the Creative Mindfulness Technique discussed in Chapter 2. Clinicians should demonstrate art mediums use prior to the client engaging in art-making to assist with creating a safe space. Art directives in the early stages of assessment and treatment planning should be well thought out providing a safe space contributing to creating the therapeutic alliance. As treatment progresses it may be fitting to choose art directives or art medium that pushes a client out of their comfort zone. Knowing when to do this varies depending on the client's experience. Pénzes et al. called the experience of clients using art materials *material interaction* (2014). The client's *material experience* as the reaction to the material on both an emotional and cognitive level trained art therapists associate to components of the client's overall mental health (Pénzes, 2014). Occasionally the clinician may need to pause the session if they see signs that the client is significantly struggling or regressing in affect and/or behavior. Some tension is helpful in treatment, but too much can result in a lapse in growth or even regression. The level of control a client desires have will impact their experience in a session regardless of what materials is provided. This need may become less rigid over time as the therapeutic alliance develops and maintains a secure environment to acquiesce to gentle experimentation which has the potential to result in flexibility, pleasure, excitement, self-efficacy, confidence, and growth in resilience (Snir, 2013; Pénzes, 2014). This is especially true when considering the process portion of a session where a client is able to explore personal meaning, thoughts, and feelings with the witness of the therapeutic alliance, the clinician. The completion of art directives will vary in length of time needed some may require one session, while others may require multiple sessions.

Multicultural Considerations and the Creative Mindfulness Technique

While art is universal, art therapists must take other factors into consideration when choosing art mediums and art directives. Some of these considerations are applied due to past trauma, while some acknowledge the many intersections one individual carries with them in their personal narrative. Some intersections bring with them the experience of marginalization. Intersections may include race, gender, sexuality, ability/disability, documentation, socioeconomic status, political views, and religious beliefs. Karcher also connects these intersections to collective trauma (2017). "Treatment needs to reactivate the capacity to safely mirror, and be mirrored, by others, but also to resist being hijacked by others' negative emotions" (van der Kolk, 2014, p. 59). A clinician's privilege may undermine the therapeutic relationship with assumptions. In order to effectively mirror a client, the clinician must take into account marginalized client's backgrounds and the impact of oppression they and their ancestors have faced (Talwar, 2010; Kapitan, 2015). Collective trauma is broader than intergenerational trauma in that it encompasses an entire group's experience or *shared injury* (Saul, 2014). Collective trauma may be caused "by disaster as well as the cumulative effects of societal oppression, poverty, displacement, and illness" (Saul, 2014, p. 1). Some factors consistently involved in trauma include not being seen, mirrored, or taken into account (Van der Kolk, 2014; Karcher, 2017).

Treatment should incorporate opportunities for these components to be addressed with care and sensitivity. An art therapist provides a space to be witnessed. The Creative Mindfulness Technique affords an integration of being in the moment with the art using reflection time and mirroring that acknowledges and honors where the client currently is and has been, including their experience of shared trauma. The material choice should be based on the client's needs and responses not on what the clinician believes they know about how art materials generally impact individuals. As noted earlier clinicians should have an ongoing practice to maintain multicultural competence, Ter Maat suggests the following self-reflective questions be "brought to light often and answered truthfully and honestly" by clinicians (2011).

- Who am I as a cultural being?
- How do I see myself in relation to the natural and spiritual worlds?
- Where am I in terms of my racial identity?
- Am I close to accepting that who I am is because of where I came from?
- Or am I questioning the attitudes and beliefs of my family or culture of origin?
- Do I think that color does not matter?
- Am I spreading cultural stereotypes, whether intentional or not?
- Where do I belong?
- With what culture, if any, do I primarily identify?
- What are my cultural norms and values (Ter Maat, 2011)?

The praxis of this ongoing work will result in the provision of a safe therapeutic antiracist space incorporating a continuous cycle of action based on reflection.

2 Mindfulness: Being in the Moment

The Unconscious

The unconscious has been a consideration in mental health treatment since its beginning with psychoanalyst Sigmund Freud. Often the unconscious refers to processes in the mind that do not come forth through intentional introspection, but come more automatically and can relate to an individual's interests. Freud saw much of this subject matter surfacing in dreams or often in slips of the tongue. Sometimes forgotten memories and motivations may also drive the unconscious (Halsey, 1977). Unlike Freud who saw his role as one to analyze the client, the approach of an art therapist is not to analyze the art.

In the beginnings of art therapy, Margaret Naumberg saw the benefits of mental health treatment undergoing analysis herself (Rubin, 2016). In her own work, she saw the value and was influenced by Freud's inclination to bring the unconscious to the surface (Rubin, 2016). Carl Jung also influenced the field of art therapy, although unlike Freud his focus was not to analyze a client. Jung believed that Freud's approach fostered an environment of dependence on the clinician. Jung sought to establish an exchange between the unconscious and the conscious seeking equilibrium and balance (Rubin, 2016). Jung regarded symbols as having an important role in self-analysis providing a great deal of hidden information. Jung also believed that all humans shared a collective unconscious including archetypes that were common in all cultures (Swan-Foster, 2016). To Jung, these symbols were potential unifiers paving the way for the psyche to resolve inner conflicts. Art was a method to work with these archetypes. Naumberg, who was personally impacted by her own experiences, went on to develop *dynamically oriented art therapy* (Rubin, 2016). Naumberg cultivated her approach around the *release* of unconscious imagery through *spontaneous art expression* (Rubin, 2016, p. 74). Naumberg ascertained the art process not only as communicative, but also as cathartic and a vehicle to express the unconscious through the art process. Additionally, Edith Kramer was a firm believer in sublimation as an appropriate and productive method of externalizing innate urges (Kramer, 1972, 1979, 2016).

DOI: 10.4324/9781003036777-2

The field of art therapy has continued to evolve and grow impacted by clinical theory's evolution, but what remains the same is that art therapists continue to foster the process by creating a safe space to create art and reflect on it. The unconscious is often tapped in this organic process providing a direct route to externalization. Spontaneous expression is any art-making without an art directive. In psychoanalytic theory, spontaneous expression is linked to free association, which is thought to provide access to the unconscious.

Be Here Now

With many uses of mindfulness in the world today, all come from the same intention of working at "accepting where one is at in their current state" (Short, 2016). Tang et al. (2015, pp. 213) define meditation as a type of training conditioned to "improve an individual's core psychological capacities, such as attentional and emotional self-regulation." Mindfulness meditation comes from the originator of Mindfulness-Based Stress Reduction (MBSR), Jon Kabat-Zinn, who defined mindfulness meditation as a process of paying attention on purpose in the moment without judgment (1994). Kabat-Zinn went on to create an eight-week systematic training program intending to teach individuals how to use mindfulness meditation to more effectively manage stress, pain, and illness (1990). While the term originates in Buddhist meditation, most cultures incorporate some form of meditation.

The benefits of meditation and mindfulness may include alleviating mental and physical conditions, though research is still in its early stages. Davidson and Kaszniak (2015) maintain that measuring the benefits of mindfulness proposes challenges due to much of the data relying on individual self-report. It has been noted that mindfulness meditation may provide a range of benefits, which may include an increase in the ability to attend to one's mental processes including managing and modulating emotions (Tang et al., 2015). Mindfulness meditation has the potential to impact our consciousness and how we experience life. While the senses are markers that trigger awareness it is impossible to incorporate every event encountered in life due to limitations in a human's capacity for attention (Csikszentmihaly, 1990, 1996). Mindfulness meditation provides an opportunity to enhance our experiences by intentionally focusing one's attention to the experience of the here and now. Csikszentmihaly saw the benefits to the integration of one's actions supporting the *flow* state, which mindfulness meditation can assist in achieving (1990, 1996). Csikszentmihaly purported a happier life for those who were able to incorporate the integration consistently (1990, 1996).

In practicing mindfulness meditation the use of the breath may be utilized as a grounding mechanism, while the individual shifts focus to the current state. Most experience moments where the mind may wander. With practice, the individual is likely to develop the ability to monitor and shift their focus to the breath when intrusive thoughts arise. This process takes practice and patience just like learning any new technique or skill. Over time the individual becomes more readily able to observe "the functioning of his or her own mind in a calm and unattached manner" (Davidson, 2015). A consistent mindfulness practice that is implemented into everyday life can result in one more consistently maintaining a relaxed brain and sense of self. "An integral part of the practice is to cultivate an attitude of kindness, acceptance, generosity, and patience toward unpleasant emotions and thoughts that may arise" (Amutio et al., 2015, p. 1572). It should also be noted that age and cultural appropriateness must be considered, as struggles are unique to each individual and the intersections that make up their life narrative.

Mindfulness and the Eight Dimensions of Wellness

Now that a basic understanding of mindfulness has been established it is critical to consider how the practice can be beneficial when incorporated throughout one's life. Doing so requires a comprehensive examination of the dimensions of wellness to provide a more accessible and outlined approach. Csikszentmihaly saw the relevance in the unification of life themes (1990). Typically, humans function in eight dimensions of wellness: they are emotions, social experiences, spirituality, intellectual functioning, the environment, the physical body, occupation/vocation, and finances. Close examination of these without impediments or distractions provides opportunities for sustainable changes and growth (Short, 2016). If a client is experiencing a depressive disorder they will likely encounter struggles in the emotions and will likely impact other dimensions potentially causing conflicts (e.g. avoiding relationships with others, poor performance at work/school, poor physical health). Incorporating the Creative Mindfulness Technique into the process of balancing the eight dimensions of wellness affords a safe and accepting structure for clients to explore and navigate life systems and patterns that may be reevaluated over treatment.

Emotional Wellness

Emotions are reactions to an experience that starts the arousal of the nervous system, including biological reactions to our mental states (Mauss et al., 2008; Short, 2016). Emotions provide individuals with sensations in the body that create both physical and psychological changes. These changes have the potential to impact thoughts and behaviors. How one emotes is impacted by many factors including but not limited to our current mood, temperament, motivation, hormones, neurotransmitters, life story intersections, and attachment. Our family culture, gender, ethnic background, and socioeconomic status also present *implicit norms* which have a significant impact on emotional wellness requiring focusing on understanding, managing, and appropriately expressing our life experiences (Mauss et al., 2008; Short, 2016). A large part of this work includes self-evaluation and self-acceptance. An individual's experience of attachment also significantly impacts their resilience, which can then impact behavior. Children typically learn at a young age how to manage frustration and employ coping skills that may involve self-soothing. If this work is not completed in childhood, resiliency is impacted resulting in maladaptive methods of emoting which last into adulthood (Malchiodi, 2012a).

Using the CMT in relation to feelings and how they are expressed provides the individual with a deeper understanding of their experience and how to navigate it. For instance, a person may endure what they call sadness, however, the emotional reaction may be due to the loss of a loved one and may be more complex encompassing a variety of feelings including loneliness, grief, and abandonment. Clarification of these more descriptive feelings can shift treatment more expeditiously creating opportunities to address specific struggles unique to each feeling. Using the CMT approach provides clients with the ability to feel more in control of their feelings during challenging times. Using mindfulness provides a place to honor the moment and fully accept what it brings.

Social Wellness

Humans are naturally social beings looking to build a sense of connection with others through belonging to and establishing strong support systems. In the year of 2020 humankind was impacted in a multitude of ways by the COVID-19 pandemic. Social distancing became a lifestyle and mask-wearing changed how we experienced facial expressions and non-verbal messages. Social wellness is contrived through casual associations, close friendships, and intimate relationships all impacted by expectations (Short, 2016). Ideals and expectations are formed at an early age in family culture and this circle grows as individuals expand social circles to playmates, friends, enemies, teachers, or strangers. Expectations become unconscious lists that are always a work in progress as one experiences rewarding moments with others or may feel let down by the action of another. Each person on the planet brings with them their unique intersections to these relationships, encountering others in a multitude of ways. However for the sake of measuring expectations in these social exchanges, one could classify any meeting into one of five categories of relationships (Short, 2016):

- **Strangers:** A relationship with anyone we do not know but share the planet with (e.g. those passed on the sidewalk, neighboring car, or in line at the grocery store). Once one crosses from a stranger to any of the other levels they cannot return to being a stranger.

- **Professional relationships:** A relationship with one who provides a professional service and has an ongoing relationship in one's life, but are not strangers (e.g. Doctors, baristas, letter carriers, therapists, teachers). Professional boundaries are practiced, often with ethical principles.
- **Shared history:** A relationship consisting of one or more shared experiences with another that may be positive or negative. Depending on the connection one may choose to nurture the attachment, which would result in the relationship moving into another category.

  - *Positive:* An exchange that is based on a positive encounter (e.g. parents chaperoning a field trip who have a pleasant exchange, high school friends who lose touch after graduation).
  - *Negative:* An exchange that holds negative undertones (e.g. cousins who have no contact as they grow into adulthood because one chooses not to be connected based on childhood bullying, a couple who separate due to one's promiscuous behavior).

- **Intentional relationships:** A relationship where one deliberately engages with another and consistently nurtures its growth. May vary in intensity.

  - *Low:* Friends with low consistency connecting, positive and somewhat superficial (e.g. old friends from college who have reconnected on social media, parents in child's school).
  - *Medium:* Friends with moderate consistency in connecting, some sharing of personal successes and struggles (e.g. monthly book club, running group).
  - *High:* Friends with high consistency connecting, sharing deeper details of daily life, and supporting each other (e.g. consistent contact, celebrate birthdays/holidays together).

- **Intimate relationships:** A relationship where there is a high level of emotional intimacy that may be shared by extremely close friends, partners, spouses, or family members. In an intimate relationship, both individuals have a high level of trust for the other, have open communication, and feel secure in their roles. This should not be confused for physical intimacy, which can be shared at other levels without emotional intimacy.

It is important to note that individuals may enter into a relationship with another and see them differently than the other sees them. One is likely to feel disappointed and potentially question if they did something wrong.

Example #1 Sam and Connor, two friends from college, had an *intimate relationship* bonding over four years of school as roommates. After graduation, Sam moved out of the country and while they stayed in touch

Sam unconsciously began to see Connor more as an *intentional relationship* with moderate consistency connecting online and rarely in person. Connor stayed in the town they went to school in and was offered a job on campus. Connor unconsciously still considered Sam an *intimate relationship* and was often disappointed at the lack of urgency Sam seemed to put forth in connecting.

Example #2 Maddie and Flora are sisters. As children, they grew up in a house full of chaos. Their father was inconsistent with his parenting sometimes creative and engaging, while others are boisterous and unpredictable. He also was somewhat controlling of their mother. Their mother was submissive and while Maddie and Flora did not see domestic violence they often experienced significant tension. Maddie, Flora's older sister by eight years, tended to Flora's needs often in an attempt to avoid their caregivers. They served as each other's mail confidant. As children, Flora and Maddie would have been in an emotionally *intimate relationship.* As an adult, Flora began counseling working through the experiences of trauma from childhood chaos, which impacted her daily functioning and relationships. While working through these struggles she attempted to discuss her realizations with Maddie who was not interested in engaging in the conversation and would only say, "the past is in the past." Over time their contact became solely around large family milestones (e.g. a family funeral) and the day-to-day diminished. As adults Flora's relationship with Maddie had transitioned to *shared history (negative type)* considering their connection was based on trauma and chaos.

In both of these examples, individuals had unmet expectations. These are not set in stone, however, while Flora's and Maddie's expectations of each other are unmet, there could be room for change depending on the engagement of each individual. "With these levels come different layers of investment in each relationship based on the priorities and expectations we have for each other" (Short, 2016, p. 33). It should be restated that the intersections a person brings with them impact each connection, although awareness is not being accountable or taking responsibility. Practicing mindfulness in social awareness provides one with the opportunity to be fully present and accepting of oneself and those around them. From here there are opportunities to connect, learn, and grow.

Spiritual Wellness

Since the dawn of humankind, individuals have looked for some meaning in life. Spirituality is a practice that is highly personal. While most automatically relate spirituality to religion, there are many ways to bring spiritual practice into daily living, by incorporating experiences or practices like private prayer, meditation, yoga, or even intentionally communing with nature. Prayer itself comes in many forms including singing, incantations, formal statements, or spontaneous verbalizations. At a deeper level, spirituality can be akin to a quest for purpose regardless of a person's chosen spiritual practice. At a deeper level, spirituality is the overarching term for one exploring personal values, morals, and integrity. Cognitive dissonance often surfaces as new information or concepts differing from pre-existing beliefs and practices are introduced (Short, 2016). In mindfulness practice, cognitive dissonance provides opportunities to explore personal awareness.

Codes of conduct can be linked to spirituality and are usually taught at a young age evolving throughout life. Lessons in morality, integrity, and tolerance come from the behaviors and reactions of others. Many religions employ storytelling to teach lessons. Many wars have been fought worldwide because of intolerance. On January 6, 2021, America watched as democracy was shaken by a violent and angry mob who charged the Capitol in Washington DC. The hoard was incited by a narcissistic leader, Donald Trump, who sat idly waiting more than six hours to address the violence resulting in five deaths. Few were arrested on the spot unlike the responses to Black Lives Matter protests around the country displaying an unequal power dynamic. Differences in consequences based on race, religion, or gender are unacceptable. Ibram X. Kendi (2019) equated racism to an addiction identifying the need for ongoing self-reflection and self-examination. The same is true for any differences that have led to unfair power dynamics in human relations. While tolerance is vital in how humans relate to each other this does not mean conversion. Individuals have free will to live their lives. "Behavior is something humans do, not races do" (Kendi, 2019, p. 102). With tolerance comes acceptance, which includes employing understanding, sympathy, and empathy even when experiencing conflicting beliefs or practices (Short, 2016).

Choosing to embrace conflict resolution and peace provides opportunities for self-examination and deep exploration around power dynamics that may violate another's rights and/or put another in danger. Employing mindfulness in spiritual practice in deepens insights on relating others using tolerance employing thoughtful and compassionate conversations and actions. "Highly compassionate people may go out of their way to physically, spiritually, or emotionally support another" (Short, 2016, p. 49). As the dimensions are interwoven, spiritual wellness heavily impacts self-concept influencing all facets of life. It is noteworthy to consider that increased compassion has bearing on thoughtfulness around equity and equality and a broadened concept of social justice possibilities providing fertile ground for enlightened interdependence in relationships also impacting social wellness.

Intellectual Wellness

Intellectual wellness incorporates curiosity, problem-solving, contemplation, and learning each of which impact other dimensions of wellness

(Short, 2016). As already stated, each person brings with them many intersections, learning styles one of them. Humans have the capacity to enhance innate abilities with continued active engagement in stimulating creative activities, critical thinking, evaluation, prediction, and comprehension. Engaging in activities that activate and increase intellectual wellness "reduces stress and increases competency in time management, listening and communication skills (both) socially and professionally" (Short, 2016, p. 63).

Critical thinking, much like mindfulness, involves deeper observation, reflection, reasoning, and communication. A clinician might explore the following steps involved in critical thinking with clients to provide structure to achieving treatment goals:

1. Recognition of the potential problem
2. Gather and interpret information
3. Explore potential assumptions or outcomes that might arise
4. Prioritize actions and methods
5. Act
6. Reflect on belief-based patterns
7. Acknowledge outcome

Through the process of employing critical thinking individual exercises their choices and beliefs, while exploring outcomes with curiosity. Individuals struggling with self-worth may find the exercise intimidating at first falling into harsh self-criticism but with support may potentially experience empowerment.

Environmental Wellness

Environmental wellness focuses on the relationships individuals have to natural environments, the places they live, work and play. These locales can be seen as an extension of the self. Using mindfulness in this dimension expands awareness of the relationship and how one's environments' impact the other life dimensions. "In developing a realistic and consistent environmental aesthetic we are able to maximize a harmonious relationship between humankind and the planet we depend upon" (Short, 2016, p. 80). Each individual impacts the planet, their community, and their immediate environment. The following true or false statements provide insights on individual environmental aesthetics (Short, 2016).

- I make an effort to refill my personal water container instead of buying plastic bottles of water.
- I make an effort to eat locally or when shopping for food purchase items considering the least amount of transportation to get my food to me.

- I turn things off and unplug them when I am not using them.
- When I can I walk, ride my bike, or use public transportation.
- I use environmentally friendly cleaning supplies.
- I have registered for paperless billing and do all bill pay electronically.
- I consistently use recycled bags for grocery shopping.
- I recycle and compost weekly.
- I do not smoke.
- I keep my living space clean consistently.

It is also vital to acknowledge that personal environmental wellness impacts each person uniquely. The items in one's home, workspace, even the inside of their car impact one's experience. Homes are decorated uniquely to interests and taste. Items used in decor may be passed down and hold personal stories of family, while some may have items purchased purely on their visual aesthetic. Items that may have been handed down through the generations come with emotional residue. Some may have positive stories, but some may have difficult stories. Clients may no longer "see" the items any longer given that the items have been in their environment for such a long period of time. Using mindfulness while evaluating the home environment will engage the senses and provide insights on items that may be best served boxed up into storage or given away completely. Using mindfulness to carefully consider one's surroundings transforms ones home into their personal sanctuary.

Physical Wellness

Physical wellness incorporates caring for the body's optimal health and daily functioning in physical activity, nutrition, and mental wellbeing (Short, 2016). Most automatically connect their physical wellness to physical weight and while this impacts health, mental welfare plays a substantial role. Benefits of engaging in consistent physical activity include reduced risk of disease and strokes, more energy, and stronger bones and muscles (Short, 2016). Many start strong and then give up, engaging in activities that are unrealistic for a sustainable practice setting one up for failure which can result in decreased self-worth. Finding the right blend of activities is vital for long-term success and will support the other components of physical wellness. Having a partner or trainer will also increase accountability and follow through. Using mindfulness during physical activity promotes a strong connection to the body, which in turn results in more focus in the moment reducing the potential for injury. "Through a consistent practice of mindfulness, you can be more in tune with your body and react to the first signs of struggles, illness, or discomfort" (Short, 2016, p. 93).

Four types of physical activity (Short, 2016):

1. **Endurance/aerobic:** This type of exercise increases breathing and heart rate and benefits the heart, lungs, and circulatory system. May include brisk walking/jogging, yard work, dancing.
2. **Strength:** This type of exercise increases muscle strength and benefits the ability to carry on in everyday activities with ease (e.g. climbing stairs, carrying groceries). May include lifting weights, resistance bands, Pilates, or using body weight/gravity in exercises.
3. **Balance:** This type of exercise decreases the potential for falls in older adults. May include standing on one foot, heel-to-toe walk, Tai Chi.
4. **Flexibility:** This type of exercise stretches muscles and helps the body stay limber and more responsive to movement. Benefits include more freedom in movement for other exercise as well as in day-to-day activities. May include yoga, Pilates.

Diet or nutrition can be loaded with triggers, which may lead to struggles with anxiety, self-loathing, and feelings of failure. Convenience and cost significantly impact food choices. Many do not have access to healthy choices living in *nutritional wastelands* (Gidney, 2015). Even schools contribute with vending machines stocked with easily accessible cheap unhealthy choices. Malnutrition occurs when individuals do not have enough to eat or do not have the right things to eat. A person can be undernourished or overnourished with the wrong nutrients. Micronutrient-related malnutrition consists of deficiencies or excesses in important vitamins and minerals (Malnutrition, 2019). Many low-income households are susceptible to food insecurity including poor nutrition and obesity due to inadequate household resources. Clinicians may suggest engagement in federal nutrition programs that are widely available and focused on improving the health and well-being of the vulnerable. In America, the Supplemental Nutrition Assistance Program (SNAP) and the Child Nutrition Programs have proven accessible and effective.

Adding mindfulness to this dimension includes intentional meal planning and preparation, as well as in-the-moment consumption. In work with clients, the focus of the word *diet* should shift to meaning fuel and nutrition versus something temporary a person does to lose weight. It would also be advised that clients work with a healthcare practitioner and/or nutritionist when working towards viable changes outside of long-existing patterns. Additionally, professionals may assist in uncovering food allergies and sensitivities, which may have contributed to historical trials. The avoidance of tobacco, drugs and excessive use of alcohol will also increase longevity. Mental wellbeing can be dramatically impacted by nutrition and physical activity. Counseling provides a safe place to explore patterns, the past, and day-to-day conflicts impacting daily functioning. Outlets for mental struggles are vital and mindfulness meditation can be a place to bring in soothing affirmations that will complement treatment.

Occupational Wellness

Occupational wellness includes work, vocation, volunteering, or school. Working with clients in this realm may involve exploring jobs versus careers. Unfortunately, not everyone is able to work at a job they find passion doing. Ideally where one works would best encompass and engage an individual's belief system, personality, values, and lifestyle. This is not always realistic, but still, a work environment should foster acceptance and tolerance. Striving for balance and fulfillment in occupational wellness involves finding rewards be it financial as well as through job satisfaction. Whether a career or a job, vocations and work environments should appreciate an individual's skills, values, and needs. Working with and connecting with others who share intersections or are like-minded in individual attitudes, way of life, and worldviews also contributes to enriching occupational wellness. Clients may need support in brainstorming opportunities (e.g. additional schooling/training, career counseling) to make sustainable changes that result in growth and fulfillment. Mindfulness work around these topics would add insights and potentially bring awareness to new possibilities. When occupational wellness is out of sync it can impact all the other dimensions.

Financial Wellness

Financial wellness can be a great source of stress resulting in increased anxiety and depression. Much like occupational wellness, clients may need outside support (e.g. financial advisor). Banks have options to support clients in all stages of financial management including credit counseling. Clients' work in session may involve exploring personal constructs of security, competency, personal credibility, and how they spend money. Additionally, exploring goals for security both short-term and long-term will help the client stay on track in creating a sustainable future. This work may include taking a deeper look at investments, which might include personal investments like education, training, and personal development. These investments will not only support financial wellness, but will also impact other dimensions with new achievements through increased knowledge, confidence, and self-worth. Adding mindfulness to financial wellness may be incorporated through thoughtful spending vs. impulsive purchases. Using mindfulness in considering how interests and beliefs impact where and how we spend our money.

The Creative Mindfulness Technique

The Creative Mindfulness Technique (CMT) combines the use of creative techniques with mindfulness activities. The process "serves to mitigate the physiological responses of the body to trauma and rework the neuro-physiological neuronal activity of the brain. This process of rewiring the neural pathways leads to adaptation and resiliency pattern identification" (Costello, 2021). This process is steeped in the Humanistic client-centered approach with a psychodynamic undercurrent. The sessions begin with an attentive check-in and from there choosing the appropriate CMT directive based on the client's needs observed from the initial consult. In sessions, the client will engage in grounding techniques that engage the senses before and after meditation if needed. Sessions also incorporate art-making in response to the meditations. After the art-making, the client and the clinician sit together witnessing the art and reflecting. With reflection comes the process where the client externally explores thoughts, feelings, or words that come to mind when they look at the art. The clinician may see symbols in the art they want to further explore with the client. This should be done once the client has already had their time to talk about their own reflections and emotional responses. The client's verbal process with clinician support is the priority. Any additional thoughts or questions from the clinician should be brought up gently without judgment. While the clinician may have conscious flags coming up in their awareness that they may want more information about it does not mean they are red flags with alarm, but flags to gather more information from the client at the appropriate time.

Bruce Moon defined responsive art-making as a response to a situation, emotion, event, or a person, "a process that involves the artist-therapist in creating artworks as a form of therapeutic intervention" (1999, p. 78). In the CMT the client makes responsive art in each session. This approach comes from a state of mind after intentional mindfulness meditation has occurred in a safe and structured setting. This state allows for the client to relinquish the potential to overthink the concept of the product and work from a spontaneous state.

The Formal Steps of CMT

1. Being in the moment: the client will choose which is best for them at the time

    1. Discussion around what they have brought in with them
    2. Short free write (e.g. the first words that come to mind)
    3. Image or word association using tools provided by a therapist

2. Grounding: the client will choose which tool is best for them in the moment (may coincide with step 1 and again after step 3 if needed)

1. Essential oils or other scented items to ground
2. Herbal tea
3. Touch (e.g. have items available which might include textured fabric, wood, stone)
4. Musical instrument (e.g. singing bowl, chime, drum)
5. Choose a color swatch to hold and look at

3. Mindfulness interventions: the client will choose which is best for them at the time

   1. Meditation activity
   2. Guided imagery
   3. Breathwork (may be used in conjunction with meditation or guided imagery)

4. Response art: the clinician will suggest art materials and directive-based on knowledge of the client's needs, struggles, strengths, and presentation after a brief check-in after the mindfulness intervention. The client will create in structured time that the therapist gently monitors

5. Reflection and process

   1. The client/artist will sit with the piece and consider the experience.
   2. The client and the therapist will explore what came up in the experience.

Alternative Supports Utilized in Mindfulness

In researching during the writing of this treatment planner supplemental supports for a mindfulness practice surfaced. Breathwork and neurofeedback could be used alone or complementary to the CMT. Some may attend weekly neurofeedback appointments in conjunction with mental health treatment. Breathwork can be a subtle but efficacious tool utilized throughout the day. What works for one person may not work for another.

Neurofeedback

Neurofeedback is a non-invasive system that is a form of biofeedback. It has been utilized in the treatment of many conditions including ADHD, stress disorders, anxiety, panic attacks, autism, depression, headaches, migraines, some types of memory struggles, and sleep disorders. During neurofeedback, EEG sensors are used to monitor brainwaves. The recipient then plays a game, listens to music, or watches a video. The process involves retraining the brain creating lasting structural changes while providing healing through neuroplasticity (Stoler, 2014). After sessions, the brain more consistently is able to operate within a more optimal range, alleviating symptoms (Stoler, 2014). At this time development, testing, and research of this approach continues to be an international effort (Hampson et al., 2020).

Breathwork

While breathwork is often a grounding tool and an undercurrent in the practice of mindfulness, it should be discussed on its own as there are a vast array of different types and traditions. Breathwork is practiced for many reasons, but similar to other mindfulness-based techniques it is difficult to track results. Some believe it boosts immunity and increases self-awareness. Some creatives tout that breathwork and meditation can aid in increasing their ability to focus on their work, enriching the creative process (Cronkleton, 2019). Many have combined breathwork and mindfulness with other treatment forms in addressing anger issues, chronic pain, depression, grief, and PTSD. Pranayama breathes in yoga is known as a controlled breathing technique that has shown an increase in the production of melatonin (Scotland-Coogan & Davis, 2016). Additionally, "improvements in autonomic functioning are seen with the long-term practice of pranayama; parasympathetic activity increases and sympathetic dominance decreases" (Scotland-Coogan & Davis, 2016).

Holotropic breathwork was developed in the 1970s by Dr. Stan Grof and Christina Grof. These group sessions conducted by a certified practitioner focus on physical, psychological, and spiritual health. Grof has described Holotropic Breathwork as a combination integrating "various elements from depth psychology, modern consciousness research, transpersonal psychology, Eastern spiritual philosophies, and native healing practices" (Grof & Grof, 2010, p. 7). Participants lie down and are guided through the sessions by a certified provider breathing at a faster rate to initiate an altered state of consciousness (Grof & Grof, 2010). Music is incorporated in the sessions, as well as *meditative art* and discussion afterward (Grof & Grof, 2010). When introducing any new treatment approach to a client, collaboration with a medical professional or certified practitioner is vital. Underlying medical conditions including pregnancy or medications may be alternatively impacted by the practice. Breathwork has been known to activate hyperventilation, which can lead to dizziness, heart palpitations, muscle spasms, cognitive changes, clouded vision, decreased blood flow to the brain, ringing in the ears, or tingling of extremities.

Part II

Applications of the Creative Mindfulness Technique

3   Application

The Creative Mindfulness Technique (CMT) can be used in the treatment of many mental health diagnoses, some comorbid. Part II of this treatment planner provides CMT therapeutic interventions that support treatment goals. These goals should be revisited throughout treatment. The art therapy process pieces provide markers in treatment to revisit with the client exploring and witnessing patterns and periods of growth. As treatment plans are unique to each client so is the application of the CMT. Part II is comprised of an overview of diagnoses with the Creative Mindfulness Technique, followed by chapters including grounding tools and interventions. Before applying the CMT to treatment it is paramount to explore how mindfulness and using a creative approach to treatment works with specific struggles.

Post Traumatic Stress Disorder

Trauma comes in many forms and its impact is contingent on each person's life narrative. These life stories include positive and difficult experiences. Traumatic experiences may relate to chaos, abuse, injury, or loss. Gerge and Pedersen relate trauma to a residual state, which follows an event or situation where repercussions exceed an individual's ability to recover regardless of personal resources no matter how accessible (2017). Trauma can stunt one's ability to use creative thinking in problem-solving making situations unmanageable. Mindfulness provides opportunities for gently honoring these conflicts. In the process of beginning to heal mindfulness allows room for creative problem solving with the support of an experienced clinician.

The diagnosis of post-traumatic stress disorder (PTSD) comes after one experiences death, be it the actual death of another or the threat of death to the self or others (American Psychiatric Association, 2013). Additional events that may result in a diagnosis of PTSD include serious injury or sexual violence. Witnessing or learning of a traumatic event that has occurred to a family member or close friend may also result in the diagnosis. Additionally, witnessing repeated or extreme trauma as a first

DOI: 10.4324/9781003036777-3

responder often leads to vicarious trauma. Types of violence may include physical, sexual, domestic, or random acts. Those in the military may also experience violence in combat. Individuals experiencing PTSD often report feelings of intense fear, helplessness, or horror. These individuals also may experience flashbacks, nightmares, and a heightened startle reflex to their environment (Jongsma et al., 2014). Often a typical reaction in coping is to intentionally avoid any type of situation that may trigger them to the trauma. Some report struggles with intrusive feelings of guilt, hyper-vigilance, and difficulties focusing.

In art therapy, the effects of trauma can be mitigated and potentially transformed often resulting in increased resiliency and more consistent use of coping mechanisms. In traditional trauma treatment Herman outlines three phases of treatment (1992):

- Phase 1: stabilization and safety
- Phase 2: trauma processing
- Phase 3: reorienting to the future and life after treatment around trauma

The expressive arts therapies provide an inimitable opportunity in trauma care where all phases of treatment often become a conduit for attachment work that may have been disrupted due to the trauma. Clients utilizing art therapy in trauma work have experienced proliferation in integration, organization, and coherence in daily functioning (Avrahami, 2006; Gerge & Pedersen, 2017).

Childhood trauma is likely to impact an individual's stress response resulting in heightened fragility later in life if left untreated. The art therapy process serves as a transitional object, as Arthur Robbins described in the object relations theory (Robbins, 1998). Much like a child has a toy or a blanket that they project their thoughts, emotions, and experiences onto, the art therapy process becomes a safe place for this projection and sublimation. Through this experience, there are activations in sensory, emotional, and kinesthetic processing that are akin to the attachment experience. Making art has been proven to aid in regulation in the left hemisphere and prefrontal cortex of the brain. This occurs through the stimulation of sensory and preverbal neural pathways (Lusebrink, 2004, van der Kolk, 2014). This creative process stimulates individuals in taking creative risks often pushing outside of their comfort zone. This undertaking can vary in approachability for each individual, but with the support of a trained and experienced clinician, the art therapy process can lead to growth in self-realization, self-esteem, and overall resiliency. Adding mindfulness to treatment provides a gentle approach and may lessen the potential for retraumatization. Growth in resiliency includes an increased ability to self-soothe and self-regulate. Additionally, in the process, an individual may also re-story their experience shifting themselves from the victim to the survivor much like in the narrative therapy approach.

Treatment of trauma must also consider the many intersections a client brings with them; some may have a place in the diagnosis. Using a lens that recognizes multicultural differences will create opportunities for clients to explore how their culture may impact the underlying conflicts. Treatment goals should focus on eliminating the negative impact the trauma-related symptoms have on all areas of client functioning. Ideally, treatment should aid in discontinuing intrusive thoughts of the traumatic experience potentially ensuing in increased interest in activities or relationships that may have been put off. Additionally, over time with treatment, the individual will be able to discuss or think about the experience without feeling physiological or psychological distress. Implementing the CMT provides a gentle and engaging structure for clients to foster creativity while experiencing healing and self-empowerment.

Anxiety

Generalized anxiety disorder (GAD) has become one of the highest diagnoses among children, adolescents, and adults. Anxiety differentiates itself from fear in that "anxiety is anticipation of future threat" (American Psychiatric Association, 2013, p.189). Many struggles accompany anxiety including excessive or possibly unrealistic worries that are difficult to control. Jongsma indicates that the individual may also experience various types of motor tension, which may include restlessness, tiredness, dry mouth, trouble swallowing, nausea, and possibly diarrhea (2014). Hypervigilance is also a common symptom and may impede focus, sleep and contribute to the individual being irritable or nervous (Jongsma, 2014). Anxiety disorders occur more often in females than males and can relate to many events in an individual's experience of life (American Psychiatric Association, 2013). For instance, anxiety in social situations may lead to avoidance of relationships to avoid negative outcomes or feeling negatively judged by others. Conversely, separation anxiety disorder occurs in relation to an individual's home or caregivers.

In the treatment of anxiety long-term goals focus on reduction of the anxiety with the treatment focus on exploring the crux of the struggle, while strengthening coping mechanisms in anticipation of abatement in symptoms. Abbing et al. suggested three different types of art-making in the treatment of anxiety; art-making as a soothing tool, art-making to express one's self, and art-making as a symbolic expression of challenging emotions and memories ensuing trauma (2018). We can speculate that art therapy may promote multiple benefits in the reduction of anxiety symptomatology. The results cannot be denied whereas they have illustrated how in the flow-like state of mind one is likely to experience a decrease in cortisol levels resulting in a decline in stress and anxiety

(Sandmire et al., 2012). Mindfulness-based training was found beneficial in the treatment of patients with fibromyalgia (Amutio et al., 2014). These patients were followed for seven weeks of treatment and training self-reporting throughout on anxiety and depression symptoms with scores significantly decreasing with additional benefits including anger control (Amutio et al., 2014). In the treatment of anxiety, adding mindfulness to the approach has the potential to extend the work beyond the therapy session where the client may continue to create a sustainable practice in their day-to-day utilizing the CMT applications to follow.

Depressive Disorders

Depressive disorders expand upon an emotional stratification with symptom combinations and severity unique to each individual. While there are many depressive disorders differentiated in the DSM-V there are commonalities amongst each. Each has "the presence of sad, empty, or irritable mood, accompanied by somatic and cognitive changes that significantly affect the individual's capacity to function" (American Psychiatric Association, 2013, p. 155). Symptoms may differ in the span of time and duration as the core struggles may have different presentations for individuals. Depressive disorders may bring with them loss of appetite and may impact the individual's desire to participate in activities they had previously enjoyed. Individuals may also experience sleep struggles, lack of energy, and complications with concentration. They may also experience feelings of hopelessness, worthlessness, or guilt impacting self-esteem. These struggles also may impact the desire to be with others resulting in withdrawal. Some also experience suicidal thoughts and/or gestures (American Psychiatric Association, 2013). Some creative mindfulness techniques to follow focus on self-concept and working with symptoms, breaking down the diagnosis into manageable pieces to integrate both in and out of the therapist's office.

The focus of treatment should mitigate symptoms to a point where the individual is able to return to a conducive level of functioning. The process should include the individual being able to acknowledge and manage feelings of depression (Jongsma et al., 2014). Goals should provide the individual with options to work on beliefs about themselves and others while examining the conflict that swayed the onset. This acceptance provides insights around patterns that could lead to relapse into a depressive episode. Goals should promote healthy interpersonal relationships, but may also need to incorporate the acknowledgment of grief if the loss is related to the core conflict. Work in this area may include an exploration around expectations and social relationships as outlined in Chapter 2.

Amutio et al. affirm that a "mindfulness practice helps patients to interrupt depressogenic reactions toward pain and other related symptoms"

(2014, p. 1572). One study found practicing mindfulness for five minutes on four occasions over a two-week period significantly improved participants' depression, anxiety, and stress levels (Strohmaier et al., 2021). In a study with medical students, researchers surmised that the mindfulness practice could potentially protect one from increased symptomatology (Alzahrani et al., 2020). Art therapy provides clients with a therapeutic relationship incorporating complex dynamics through the application of the art process. The clinician must be equipped to hold a safe space with patience providing space and time for clients to process the art to the fullest and remain engaged in all the phases in the treatment of depression. Depressive disorders can be all-encompassing with often painstakingly slow changes. A clinician must work with gentle consistent presence, supporting and witnessing treatment, "we must truly know the person with whom we are working, and persistently, delicately, and compassionately assist in pushing back the dark" (Wise, 2015, p. 359). Many have discontinued treatment when not feeling aligned with their provider at times with critical life-threatening outcomes.

Grief

Grief can be debilitating. Loss may be unexpected or anticipated through illness and deaths or grief may stem from life transitions that also may have been unexpected or anticipated (e.g. moving, job loss, termination of relationship). Some feel the guilt associated with their loss and if the triggering event is related to transition one may be without a support system to manage through their struggles. Grief is expressed differently by individuals due to age, past experience, and culture. Kübler-Ross developed the stages of grief as denial, anger, depression, bargaining, and acceptance (1970). These stages aren't experienced in a linear fashion; an individual may bounce between them experiencing some more than once.

The grief experience for children may involve emotional shock, regressive behavior, mood swings, and while they may be living in a home where multiple family members are experiencing grief, they may not be involved in serious decisions or receive information that adults may deem as inappropriate for them. Due to immature cognitive development, some children do not understand the loss as irreversible. Children also often have a limited capacity in verbalizing and tolerating emotional pain. Engaging in mindfulness with children in relation to grief and loss would be best focused on self-regulation and self-soothing. Treatment for anyone should involve exploring how the grief has impacted daily life to begin the healing process (Jongsma, 2014). Clinicians must provide sensitivity and caretaking into account individual or family cultural and spiritual beliefs when supporting clients who are grieving. Many experience symptoms of depressive disorders which may abate with treatment as clients resolve feelings around the loss and begin to reinvest in daily life and relationships.

Mindfulness provides a place to process the stages of grief bringing with its acceptance that activates the parasympathetic system, the area of the autonomic nervous system that engages energy conservation, rest, and digestion (Manteau-Rao, 2016). A mindfulness practice contributes to the self-empowerment of individuals experiencing bereavement through the reduction of overwhelming and ruminating thoughts (Feng-Ying et al., 2019). In one study on bereaved individuals, participants practicing mindfulness techniques experienced an increase in consistent emotional regulation in daily functioning (Feng-Ying et al., 2019). This led to an increase in the participant's ability to relax leading to improved sleep, which translated to more vitality in their days (Feng-Ying et al., 2019). Mindfulness has also been utilized in working with the caregivers of family members with Dementia to work through pre-death grief as well as the daily stressors of providing immediate care (Manteau-Rau, 2016; Jain et al., 2019). Implementing art therapy in the grief process provides a place to dialogue with the pain. Art provides a place outside of the body to explore the reality of the loss along with the range of emotions associated with it. It also provides a safe place to emotionally relocate the deceased individual if the grief is related to death. Having visual representations supports meaning reconstruction or changing the narrative. Creative mindfulness techniques provide an opportunity to gain these positive outcomes through mindfulness meditation, while the art therapy portion provides concrete visual representations of the use throughout the grieving process.

Low Self-esteem

Low self-esteem is comorbid with many diagnoses. Often those experiencing low self-esteem have a negative view of themselves, often seeing themselves as unattractive, worthless, an encumbrance, and insignificant. These individuals often accept blame easily and conversely struggle with accepting compliments. Some who experience low self-esteem have experienced significant trauma and abuse in their childhood (Hartz & Thick, 2005). They may also be easily taken advantage of due to having poor boundaries with others for fear of rejection. Poor hygiene and awkwardness in social situations may also prevail. Goals in treatment include working towards cultivating a more consistent and positive self-image that in leads to individuals engaging in social situations without hesitation displaying a more assertive air. This work includes establishing consistent positive hygiene and self-care habits, which foment self-acceptance and self-love. Art therapy has proven effective in raising the self-esteem of female juvenile offenders (Hartz, 2005). Work with these clients provided opportunities at building connections with others as well as experiencing feelings of mastery relating to art-making.

Adding mindfulness in the treatment of low self-esteem could be seen as a form of submersion where the client intentionally practices unconditional acceptance towards themselves, feelings, and thoughts. As with any approach, the structure provided by the clinician must evoke feelings of safety. Through the non-judgmental approach, the individual becomes empowered to challenge critical thoughts about themselves (Thompson & Waltz, 2008; Randal et al., 2015). Mindfulness practice can lower levels of social anxiety (Rasmussen & Pidgeon, 2011). With ongoing practice individuals are able to cultivate and eventually maintain their attention on the present reducing sensitivity and self-criticism, separating thoughts as "mental processes rather than facts" (Randal et al., 2015). While creative mindfulness techniques provide a container to reflect on over time, one cannot deny the benefits to one's confidence associated with experimentation and possible mastery of the art techniques.

Addiction

Addiction can impact an individual biologically, psychologically, socially, and economically. Addiction is a chronic disease that transforms a person's brain functioning and changes their perception. While many only connect substances to addiction, compulsive behaviors like gambling, overeating, sex, Internet use, pornography, and shopping are also included. Individuals suffering with addiction find themselves unable to stop or cut back exposure to their focus of addiction regardless of internalized or externalized intentions. Many who grapple with addiction eventually face problems in relationships, physical wellness, their work, and may end up facing legal penalties. Over time substance use can boost tolerance levels, requiring more of the substance to obtain the coveted effect. Individuals may also exhibit physical symptoms upon withdrawal from use.

The treatment of addiction requires patience and commitment. Many rely on the *12 Steps of* Alcoholics Anonymous for structure in their journey to sobriety (Bill, 1939). The ultimate goal in recovery is focused on establishing and maintaining sobriety. Art therapists may have to modify art directives specific to treatment settings and curriculum already in place (Schmanke, 2015). Treatment involves a commitment to acquiring and maintaining the skills necessary for sustainable sobriety. Many approaches involve cognitive-behavioral techniques, additionally, shame theory can be valuable considering many fighting addictions also feel self-critical internalizing feelings. Addiction becomes a coping mechanism to mask or numb feelings that are uncomfortable to address. Mindfulness-based therapies can be extremely soothing and centering to clients suffering with addiction. Clients with pornography addiction have experienced an increase in personal awareness of thoughts, emotions, bodily sensations, and behavior providing opportunities for them to explore and challenge formerly held beliefs and judgments (Fraumeni-McBride, 2019).

Art therapy is an effective approach in dealing with shame reduction. An experienced clinician is required as the art process can be a gateway flooding the client with emotional conflicts and pain. One struggling with addiction is likely to have an array of defenses in place to fall back on. Art therapy provides a safe space for nonverbal action where one can access and contain historical and present struggles using sublimation and projection in their process (Wilson, 2012). Hanes used self-portraits while working with clients and addiction and saw the portraits as an opportunity for the clients to come "face-to-face with their addictive nature" (2007). He saw the work as an opportunity for clients to work with their defense mechanisms outside of themselves, which provided a clearer view of a sense of self that had become distorted by the addiction (Hanes, 2007). Chapter 8 provides directives to work with the conflict while exploring the impact it has had on themselves, their environment, and their relationships. Schmanke described art therapy as a method of *bypassing resistance* commonly encountered in the treatment of addiction where through the process a client is able to experience and encounter emotional and spiritual meaning in their lives (Schmanke, 2015). As clients engage in art therapy they begin to accept the process of working without inhibition and develop trust in themselves. Adding mindfulness and the opportunity to accept one's self unconditionally has the potential to lead to self-actualization.

4   Art Journaling

Art journaling is a method to provide structure to treatment outside of the therapy office. Why add art to the journaling practice? One study found more short-term mood repair through art-making overwriting (Drake et al., 2011). In the creative mindfulness technique, clients may write or create art in art journals. The journal itself becomes a holding space where clients can externalize and track struggles. Art journals can also be a container for thoughts and feelings in the unconscious (Sackett & McKeeman, 2017). Art journaling may provide space for documenting the implementation of new skills acquired through treatment, but art journals are also a place to explore thoughts, behaviors, and emotions that may be associated with struggles in real-time as they occur. Art journals are a valuable tool in treatment providing a place to externalize self-talk that can be further examined in sessions where the clinician may provide feedback and support around distorted thought patterns. The clinician and client may then together delve into thoughts that are more reality-based processing potential outcomes in situations in the safe structure of the therapeutic alliance. Art journals can also be a place to document successes. Art journals are not just for clients, many clinicians also find them extremely helpful as a place to contain process art outside of sessions but influenced by clients or session contents. Clinicians have reported reduced symptoms of vicarious trauma increasing receptivity to positive experiences outside of work (Gibson, 2018).

Journals are available with many options of paper style, size, and binding. Art journals can also be handmade books or altered books as discussed in Part I. Clients should be encouraged to work freely in the process from drawing, to writing, to mixed media work depending on what feels like the right fit at the moment. In this section, the following art journal prompts can be utilized by any client if fitting to treatment goals. In the session, an art therapist may use specific art directives in sessions to further delve into content evoked by an art journal entry. The art journaling process provides opportunities to review and reinforce gains while working with obstacles.

DOI: 10.4324/9781003036777-4

Eight Dimensions of Wellness

Rationale: Individuals may engage in creating entries around ongoing struggles or processes when focusing on balancing the dimensions of wellness. Entries may focus on one or all at once and should explore conflict (e.g. anxiety, grief, trauma, depression, addiction) in real-time providing concrete information for in-session work. Entries may be a written passage or full collage. In art therapy, the visual record can be a helpful reminder to revisit when working through triggers that have been quelled in the past. Figure 4.1 depicts response art in an art journal created by a cisgender adult female.

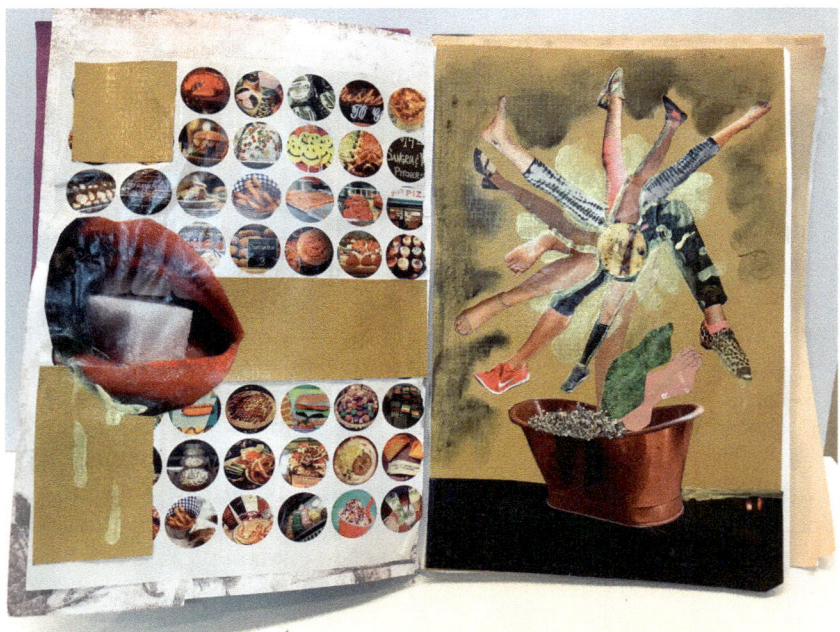

Figure 4.1 Eight dimensions of wellness.

Gratitude

Rationale: Ongoing entries on gratitude can provide a continuing marker of positive emotions, people, events, and objects. This list can be simple (e.g. coffee), complex (e.g. the singing voices at church). This entry can be any length from a few words or a picture to start the day. Entries may be a written passage or full collage. In art therapy, the visual record can be a helpful reminder to revisit when conflicts arise (Figure 4.2). With the

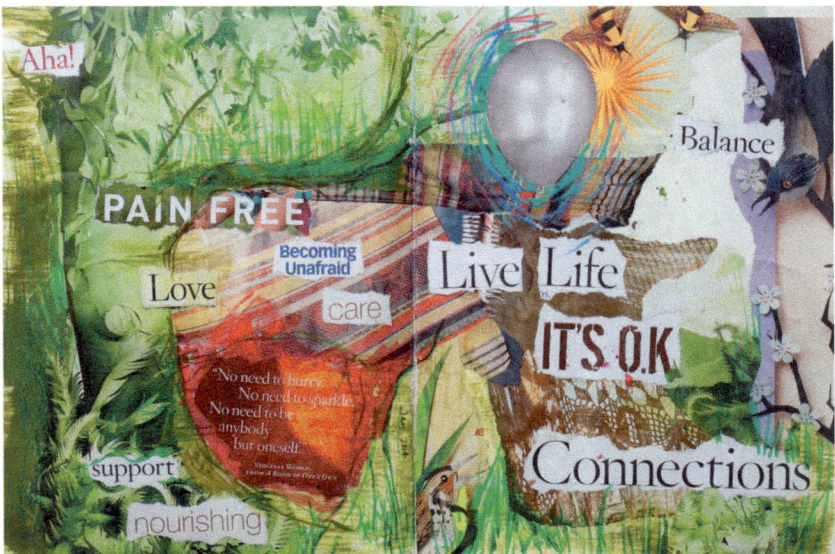

Figure 4.2 Gratitude journal entry.

CMT clients should be encouraged to use the images when engaging in grounding moments outside of sessions.

Feeling Check In

Rationale: Ongoing entries around feelings provide a place for cathartic expression in the moment. Figure 4.3 shows a mixed media piece created after mindfulness meditation. Clinicians should provide a feelings chart to clients to assist in the identification and labeling of emotions as they arise outside of sessions. This will aid in understanding triggers as they occur. These entries can be any length from a few words or a picture to a written passage or full collage. Clients may use this as an opportunity to self-monitor thoughts, feelings, and actions and share later in session with a clinician. This entry could also be expanded upon with "I" statements as discussed in Chapter 7.

Figure 4.3 titled "A Question of Moods" was created by a two-spirit Anglo/Native American individual. The piece evokes loneliness, questioning, despondency, and disempowerment which the artist confirmed feeling, but then described how the art process makes art with the "broken pieces" of the heart.

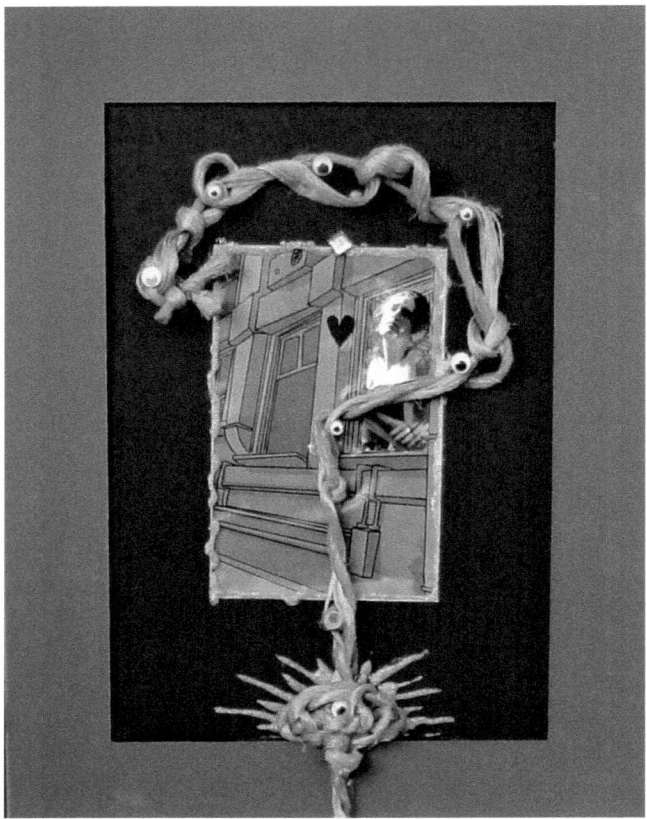

Figure 4.3 "A Question of Moods".

Self-talk

Rationale: Ongoing art journal entries externalizing self-talk messages provide opportunities to explore fear-based internalized thoughts and biases while exploring alternatives. The process with the clinician should support the client as they review and celebrate successes. In the session, the process should include assisting the client in developing positive self-talk and reframing negative self-concepts. The art journal will create a place for clients to track and identify moments when negative beliefs or thoughts are triggered. Clients may also use their art journals to create an entry honoring one positive trait or action about themselves one time daily. This may be a concrete trait (e.g. physical appearance, good cook) or more abstract traits (e.g. sound of their laughter, how they felt about a choice they made). In session process will reinforce clients' accomplishments, increasing confidence (Figure 4.4).

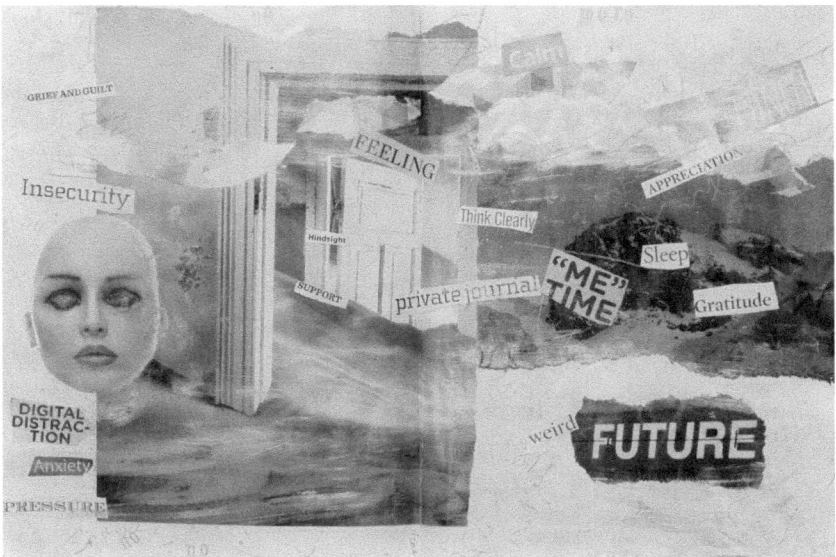

Figure 4.4 Self-talk journal entry.

From Worry to Relaxation

Rationale: Ongoing entries focused on options to refer to when feeling anxious or stressed from struggle (e.g. anxiety, grief, trauma, depression, addiction). This personalized list (words and images) should be composed of options to refer to when in conflict. The process with the clinician should also include support on incorporating and maintaining self-regulation by recognizing the moment conflict arises and then shifting to relaxation skills. Figure 4.5 illustrates response art created in a journal by a cisgender adult female.

Ritual

Rationale: This directive provides the client the opportunity to create their own rituals that may support them in their work. This will provide time and place to honor, but allow for the client to move on outside of the time-limited period (e.g. death/grief: dress in dark colors, light a candle on the anniversary of loss). Clients should be encouraged to rely on their spiritual faith as a derivation of support. Rituals may include but are not limited to prayer, meditation, worship, music, and witnessing nature. In-session follow-up and process may include exploring time limits that feel

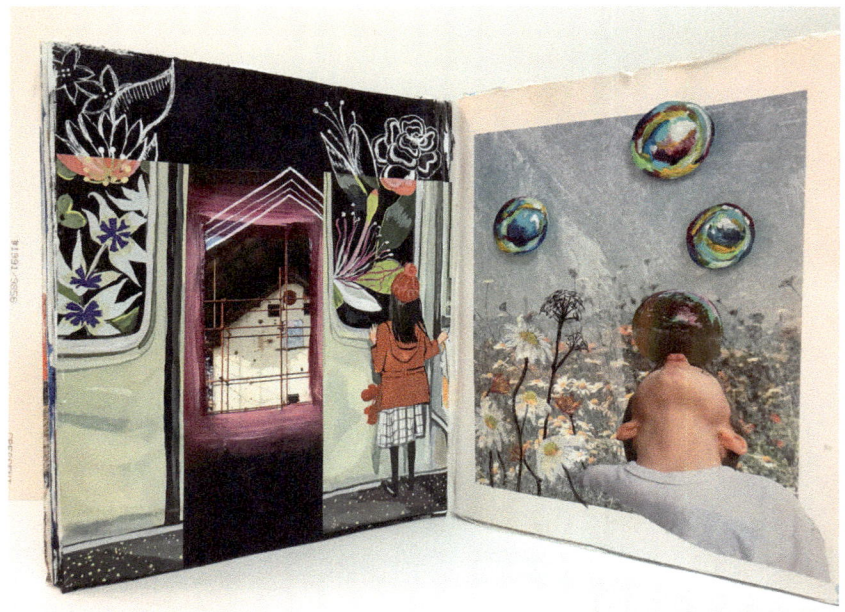

Figure 4.5 Journeys.

appropriate to the client, but not excessive resulting in regression in other areas of the 8 dimensions of wellness. Allowing the client room to create their own rituals affirms their thoughts and opinions reducing potential feelings of guilt. Figure 4.6 displays an art journal prompt was created by a white cisgender female in response to systems of self-care.

Strengths

Rationale: Ongoing entries relating to strengths from the beginning of treatment on. In session process should witness successes, reinforcing clients' growth and increasing confidence. The verbal process may include confronting negative self-talk and generating realistic self-talk. This directive will work towards challenging distorted thinking and building resilience.

Supporting the 12 Steps

Rationale: Clients may use their journals to work on the *12 Steps* addiction by doing daily pages (Alcoholics Anonymous World Services,

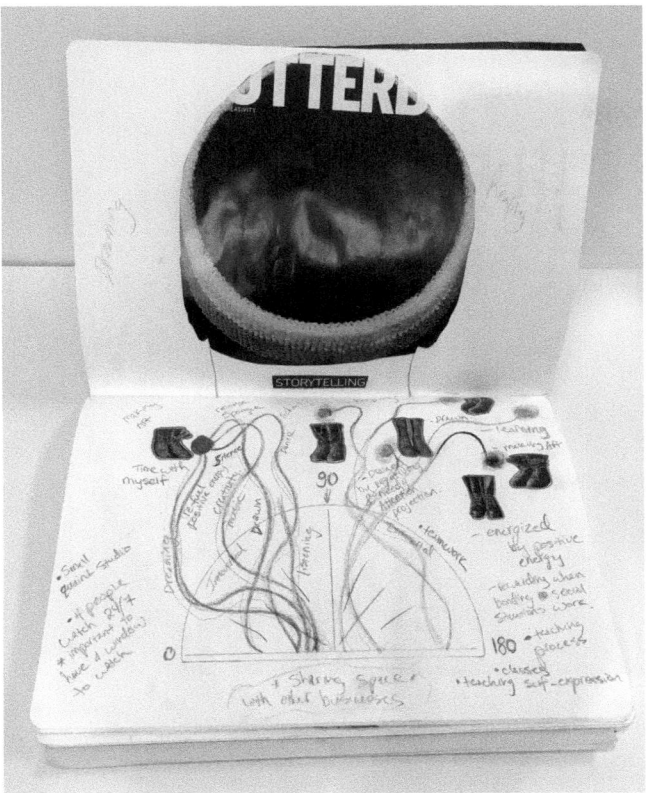

Figure 4.6 Self-care rituals journal entry.

Inc., 1989). An application of the 12 Steps might include the following mindfulness prompts and then creating art in response to them.

1. Consider the feelings of accepting the powerlessness you feel over your addiction.
2. Reflect on how spirituality impacts you.
3. Consider how it feels to let go of the things you can not control.
4. Reflect on your morals past to present.
5. Consider the feelings of admitting mistakes.
6. Consider that you are able to change who you are.
7. Reflect what it feels like to not be alone.
8. Consider those you have harmed and how to make amends.
9. Reflect on apologies you have made and received.
10. Reflect on natural consequences and choices (Figure 4.7).

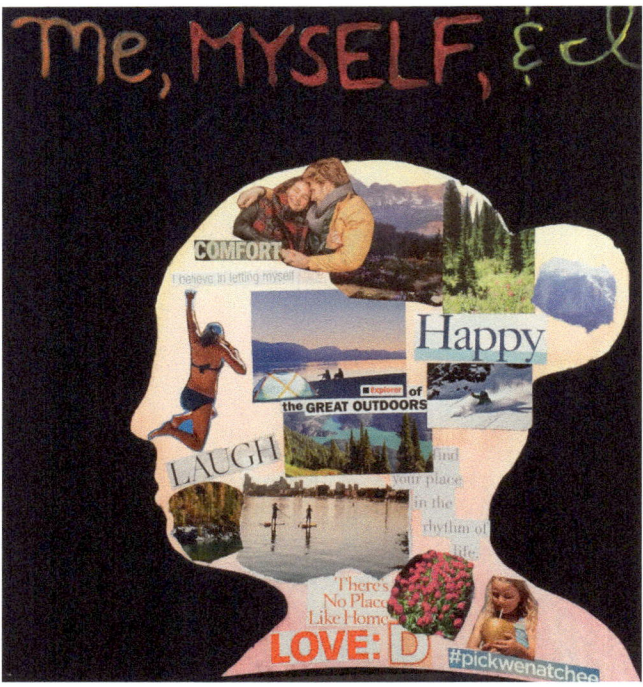

Figure 4.7 Strengths.

5 Guided Imageries

Using guided imagery in session provides the client with access to visual imagery they had not accessed in the past. During guided imagery, the client closes their eyes if they feel comfortable and then the clinician reads a guided imagery script or speaks from memory directing the client to focus on the therapist's voice and use their imagination to visualize the experience their therapist is providing. Some guided imageries may take a client to a place in their imagination while others may focus on providing the client with an experience in the body heightening mindfulness and self-awareness. Guided imageries are often helpful for individuals in the early stages of their meditation practice. Having the structure of another's voice or music can improve focus on the moment and help break from intrusive thoughts. Outside of sessions clients may access meditation applications via the Internet, some have low or no-cost options.

After the guided meditation the therapist and client process the experience with the client describing important takeaways (e.g. symbols, images, sensations in the body which may include temperature, colors, or textures). Guided imageries may be used in the creative mindfulness technique as outlined in Chapter 2.

Guided Imagery Example 1 Body Scan

This guided imagery should be read slowly with ample pauses in each area of the body. Run time 7–12 minutes. After this piece the client may work on a body outline (Figure 5.1), making response art to areas in the body they felt especially connected or disconnected to. A body scan is extremely effective in working through sleep struggles, but also a good start to the day upon waking that aids in connecting deeply with the body consistently.

When you are ready, close your eyes. Take a moment and be in your seat. Let your shoulders drop. Let your feet rest each one flat on the floor. Let your spine gently stack and your sit bones feel gravity holding you gently and safely onto your chair. Shift your awareness to your breath. Let it just be at its normal pace and rhythm. When you feel ready take a few deeper breaths, letting the exhale have noise. Feel the clean air enter

DOI: 10.4324/9781003036777-5

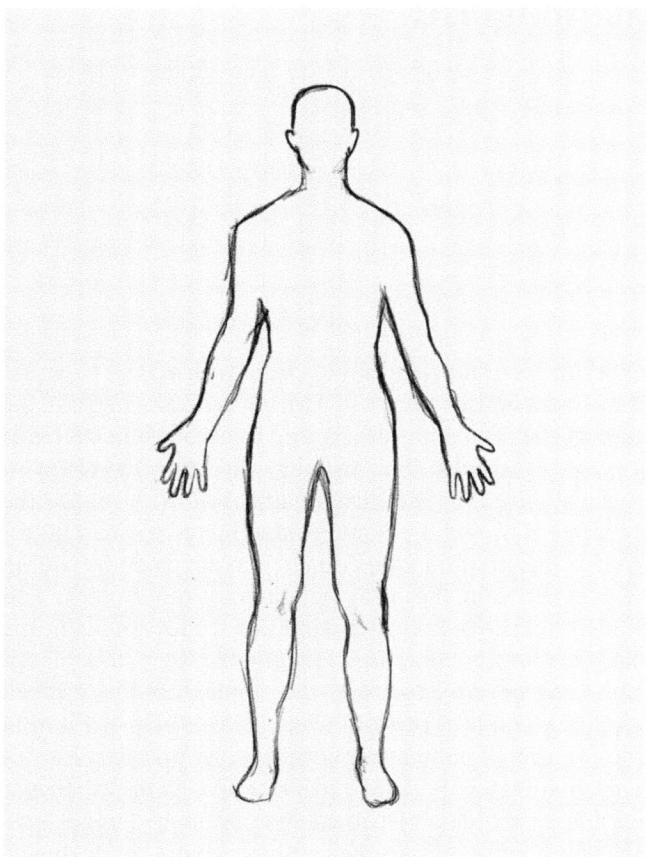

Figure 5.1 Body outline.

your body...then let the air from your lungs escape. After a few of these breaths let your breathing return to its normal rhythm.

At this time, we are going to shift your focus down to your feet. Be in your feet. Feel them resting flat on the ground. Feel the earth's gravity gently holding them to the earth. Maybe you even feel vines growing out of them into the earth below you. Notice every bone, move through your toes...to the many bones in your feet, your feet that take you so many places every day. Slowly move through your feet, to your heels, and then your ankles and then move up the lower halves of your legs, through your shins, the bone...the muscle to your knees. Rest in your knees. Imagine love and light in your knees. Be in the place where the bones come together. Notice your knees, the muscle, the tendons, the bones, and then slowly begin to move up your thighs. Through the bone, the muscle. Then rest in your sit bones. Feel the seat holding you safely and gently in earth's gravity. Be in your hips. Imagining love and light in your hips as you slowly move through your abdomen and then your internal organs, resting in your lungs. Feel the air in your lungs. Coming in bringing fresh clean to your body, then escaping out through your nose. Be in your lungs feeling the natural rhythm of your breath. Imagine love and light in your lungs. From then shift to your heart. Be in your heart. Feel your heartbeat. Imagine the blood moving in and out, receiving oxygen, and sending its nutrients to all the parts of your body. Be in your heart. Imagine love and light in your heart.

When you are ready shift your attention to your shoulders. Splitting from your heart, into each shoulder. Feel where your arms are attached. Let the weight of your shoulders fall. Slowly move your attention down each of your arms, through the bone...through the muscle. Pausing in each elbow, then moving through each of your forearms to your wrists. Feel the space where your hands are attached and then be in your hands. Your hands with so many bones. Through your palms and into your fingers up to each fingertip. Your hands do so many things for you every day. Breathe love and light in your hands. When you feel ready you will move your attention back up through your arms, slowly, back through your wrists, elbows, biceps shoulders...back but meeting in your neck. Pause here. Be in your neck. This small opening so vital to your survival. Passage for nutrition, air...your voice. Be in your throat. Breath love, energy, and light in your throat.

When you are ready you will move up, imagine yourself climbing up into that space behind your eyes. Slowly, move into that space. Here you will have a few moments of silence to be in this space (1–3 minute pause depending on the individual). As we get close to the end of this experience the last place you will visit was a place you wish you had more time... what part of your body needs more attention? Go there now and breathe more love, energy, and light in that space (1-minute pause depending on the individual). We have come to the end of this journey through the body. When you feel ready notice the sounds outside of you (verbalize any noise in the room e.g. clock ticking, meditation music). When you feel ready open your eyes and come back to the room. Figure 5.2 was created by a cisgender young adult female during a mindfulness work-shop in response to the body scan-guided imagery. This individual used mixed media in her process.

Figure 5.3 titled *The Center of My Uterus* was created by a two-spirit Anglo/Native American adult during a mindfulness workshop. The individual reported the body scan felt timely in preparing for and mourning the impending loss of their womb from cancer surgery. They reported that the piece illustrated the "input from the universe" they saw the creative process as nurturing.

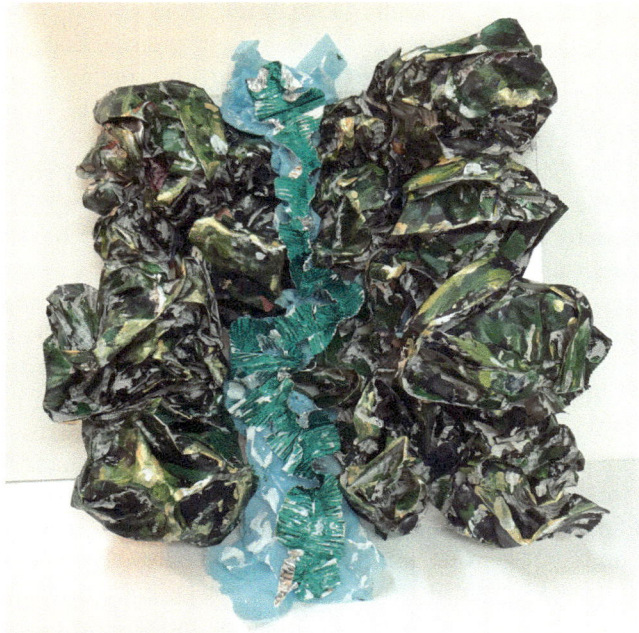

Figure 5.2 Body scan response art.

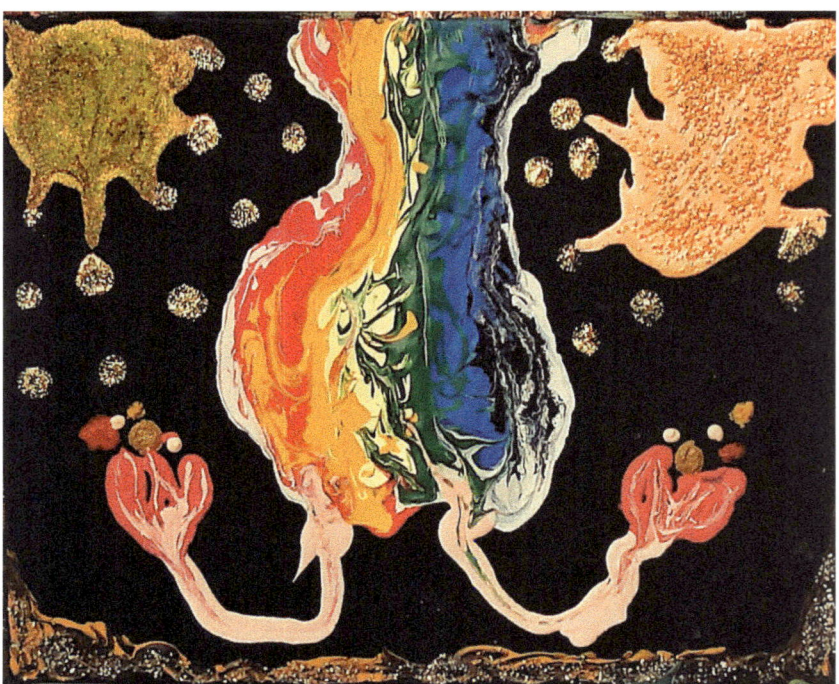

Figure 5.3 The Center of My Uterus.

Guided Imagery Example 2 Variation on an Energy Ball

This guided imagery needs to be read slowly with many pauses providing ample time for the full experience. It should take anywhere between 3–6 minutes.

When you are ready, close your eyes. Take a moment and be in your seat. Let your shoulders drop. Let your feet rest each one flat on the floor. Let your spine gently stack and your sit bones feel gravity holding you gently and safely onto your chair. Shift your awareness to your breath. Let it just be at its normal pace and rhythm. When you feel ready take a few deeper breaths, letting the exhale have noise. Feel the clean air enter your body...then let the air from your lungs escape. After a few of these breaths let your breathing return to its normal rhythm.

Now raise your bent arms letting your palms face each other shoulder's distance apart. Let your shoulders drop. Shift your focus from your shoulders moving down into each of your arms through the bone and muscle...past your elbows...through your forearms and wrists resting in your hands. Be in your hands. Imagine the energy in your palms extending into each finger. Now we are going to shift our focus from our hands to space between. Breath into that space between. Slowly move your hands just slightly together...don't rush...but continue to focus your attention on the space between. Breathe into that space. Continue. Don't rush. Inch by inch pause in between...continue to focus on that space in between. What does that space look like? What does it feel like? Pause at times...feel the energy between. Continue to slowly move them together. Remember to breathe, let that breath flow into your hands and into that space between. Eventually, your hands will come together. Let them touch. Pull them in front of your chest and rest there. Take a few more breaths imagining light, energy, and love in your hands. When you feel ready notice the sounds outside of you (verbalize any noise in the room i.e. clock ticking, meditation music). When you feel ready open your eyes and come back to the room.

Figure 5.4 depicts response art created by a nonbinary adult person of color (BIPOC) after this guided meditation through telehealth. Afterward, the client reported the sensation made them feel "stronger than you think inside."

Figure 5.5 was created by a cisgender young adult female in a creative mindfulness workshop. Participants engaged in two meditations on body scan and the other the Energy Ball. Spent the session using mixed media creating two pieces that had very unique properties in how they felt when compressed between the hands. She indicated that she wanted them to feel like her meditation experience.

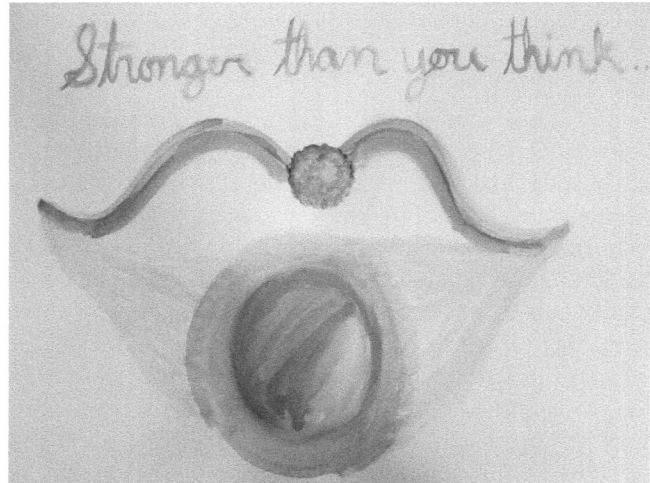

Figure 5.4 Energy ball response art 1.

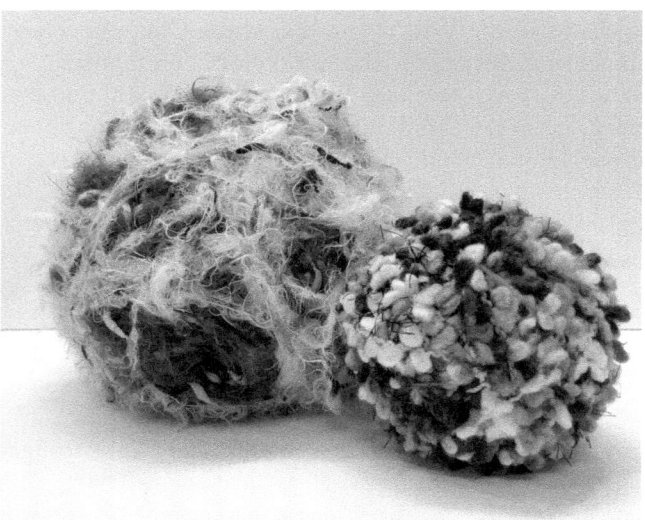

Figure 5.5 Energy ball response art 2.

Guided Imagery Example 3 Safe Place in Nature

This guided imagery should take anywhere between 5–15 minutes. It is important to instruct the client ahead of time that during this visualization they will imagine walking on a safe journey in nature but to remain seated throughout the experience.

When you are ready, close your eyes. Take a moment and be in your seat. Let your shoulders drop. Let your feet rest each one flat on the floor. Let your spine gently stack and your sit bones feel gravity holding you gently and safely onto your chair. Shift your awareness to your breath. Let it just be at its normal pace and rhythm. When you feel ready take a few deeper breaths, letting the exhale have noise. Feel the clean air enter your body...then let the air from your lungs escape. After a few of these breaths let your breathing return to its normal rhythm.

Imagine that you are sitting on a park bench. It is a warm day, but not too warm. You are comfortable and the sun is not overbearing. You see a trail not far from you and decide to go for a walk on it. Imagine standing up and walking across the sidewalk in front of you to a path that has been created into a wooded area. You feel safe and secure. You feel a familiarity and confidence to move forward. As you begin to walk on the natural path that has been created, you feel the soft ground underfoot and smell the woody air. Birds chirp and look on as you make your way down a slight slope. You begin to hear the trickle of water and decide to follow the sound. There are wildflowers along the walkway and you notice the smell of damp moss. Purple, yellow, and pink flowers sprinkled about directing your journey. Ahead you see a small stream. The soft and steady water laps onto the rocks along the stream bed. You notice the path leads to a small ancient-looking stone bridge. You continue to follow the path and as you approach the bridge you notice an old sign, but the writing is illegible. A soft wind comes from behind you, gently nudging you forward. The warm sun peaks through the leaves of the trees around you, gently warming your face. As you cross the bridge you are surprised at the craftsmanship. The ancient-looking stones rest firmly together, creating a solid base. You move across the bridge and catch the scent of a citrusy pine smell. The trees are tall and seem like guardians. On the other side of the bridge, the path resumes and winds up a small incline. The trees seem to be getting further apart and the sun up ahead illuminates a wide meadow opening. As you step into the meadow see an ocean of wildflowers of pink, blue, white, purple, and yellow. In the center, the flowers seem to have left space for you. As you move closer and closer to the center you realize that there is a blanket laid out for you. On it sits a wooden box. You sit down on the blanket and take in space, surrounded by the flowers...and then you decide to open the box.

Be there in that space. Let your breath flow naturally. Feel the temperate sun on your face. Feel the gentle breeze in the air and look at the contents of the box. In a moment you will leave the place. Take a moment to absorb all that surrounds you (provide a long pause, at least 1 minute). When you are ready come back to the room.

Figure 5.6 was created by a queer gender fluid BIPOC individual and illustrates what this client described as being "inside the box." They

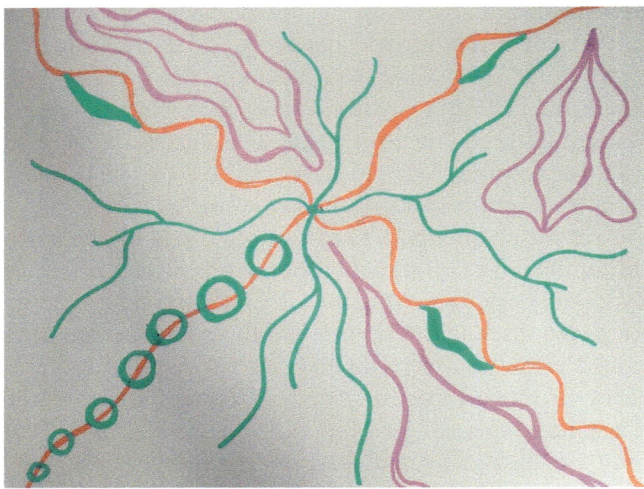

Figure 5.6 Safe place response art.

reported that initially they felt fear in the box, but then it transformed into something like space with moving balls and colors.

Guided Imagery Example 4 Inner Plant

When you are ready, close your eyes. Take a moment and be in your seat. Let your shoulders drop. Let your feet rest each one flat on the floor. Let your spine gently stack and your sit bones feel gravity holding you gently and safely onto your chair. Shift your awareness to your breath. Let it just be at its normal pace and rhythm. When you feel ready take a few deeper breaths, letting the exhale have noise. Feel the clean air enter your body...then let the air from your lungs escape. After a few of these breaths let your breathing return to its normal rhythm.

Now we will shift our focus to our seat. Be in your seat. Feel earth's gravity gently cradling you. Your sit bones support your spine as it stacks up to your skull. Be in your abdominal area. Breathe light and energy and love into your internal organs. Now imaging a small seed there. Gently glowing from your inner light. See the seed, notice its color, texture, and size...and know that it is a part of you. Send love into this precious little seed. Breathe light and energy and love into this seed. Notice that it is beginning to move and change...a small sprout of you has popped out and it is slowly reaching up while your tiny roots are growing underneath it. Watch and witness the seed as it grows slowly and gently, moving through you, your ribs lovingly protecting your chest, lungs, and heart. The plant continues to grow. Witness it moving down your arms and moving up into your head, where it has turned into a bud. The bud is growing in size that eventually begins to open into a beautiful blossom. Witness this blossom. Breathe light, energy, and love into the blossom and take a couple of minutes to be here witness to this beautiful part of you (*1–2 minutes pause depending on the individual*).

Now we have come to the point where we will return back to the room. Remember the blossom…the plant. Breathe. When you feel ready notice the sounds outside of you (verbalize any noise in the room i.e. clock ticking, meditation music). When you feel ready open your eyes and come back to the room.

Figure 5.7 was created by a queer gender fluid **BIPOC** individual during a telehealth session. They participated in the mindfulness meditation and while making art was focused on the pain they were experiencing in their body. The client identified the area in the center as being "a bit tortured."

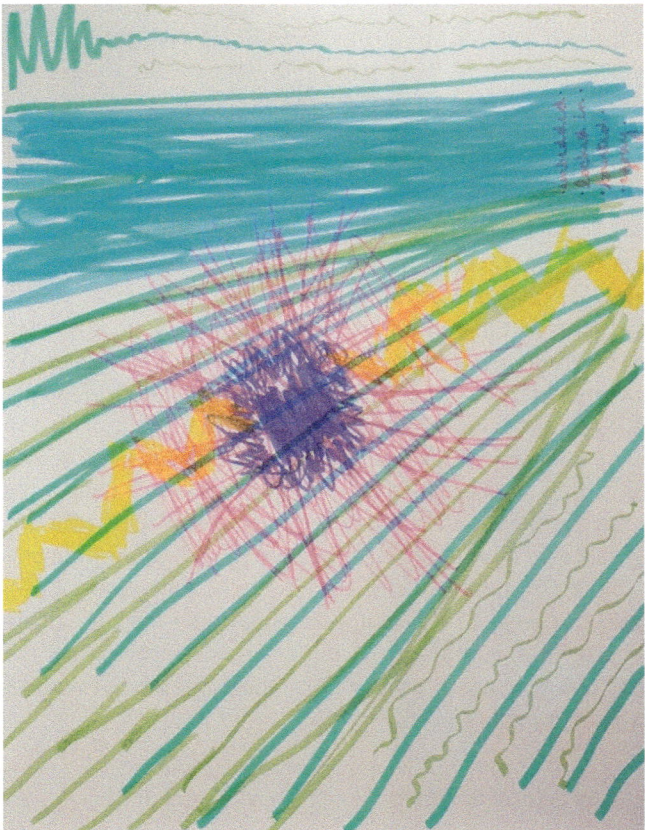

Figure 5.7 Inner plant response art.

6 Tools for Safety

Trauma-informed care supports all areas of the brain, ensuring that they remain connected to each other working in symbiosis. Tools that may be used both in and outside of treatment provide opportunities for continual restoration, especially when used in response to trauma survival reactions or defense mechanisms (Clark et al., 2014). Typical trauma defense mechanisms include *attachment cry*, *flight and fight*, *freeze*, and *collapse or feigned death* (Clark et al., 2014). An individual may make an *attachment cry* when they are in a state of hyperarousal or panic when they would typically cry out for help. When in *flight or fight* the individual's body is activated and ready for action. An individual in a *freeze* state is arrested in their ability to move and feels frozen or stuck. Lastly, in *collapse of feigned death*, the individual is completely shut down in a corpse-like state.

Psychoeducation is a key component in evidence-based mental health treatment providing clients and those they love with resources to employ when triggered. For all involved in treatment, psychoeducation promotes feelings of normalization and empowerment. Psychoeducation involves identifying triggers and then working with the client to identify the triggers as they come to recognize when the aforementioned defense mechanisms are activated (Clark et al., 2014). Having tools to engage with as triggers arise can reduce the severity of the trauma response and alleviate the intensity of the typical affective experience, while also increasing resiliency through self-empowerment, therefore, making self-regulation more efficient (Pascual-Leone et al., 2016). This chapter includes a variety of tools that aid in managing through a triggering event both inside and outside of the therapy session. Over time the implementation and consistent use of tools such as these can lessen events of dissociation and provide a marker of progress.

Creative Mindfulness Mantra Cards

Rationale: Clients may work on these inside or outside of the session. Clients will rework an old deck of cards or start with a blank deck. Clients will use words and images creating cards specific to coping strategies, affirmations, or identifying positive coping statements. Statements can be

DOI: 10.4324/9781003036777-6

personalized depending on treatment goals. Lamination also creates a lasting tool that is easy to transport in a pocket or wallet. These cards can provide comfort during difficult moments. Creating the cards provides the client with the ability to make personalized commitments to the self becoming mini contracts. In the session, these cards provide opportunities to explore diagnosis and the impacts. Figure 6.1 depicts examples of Creative Mindfulness Mantra cards on a blank deck using collage and paint.

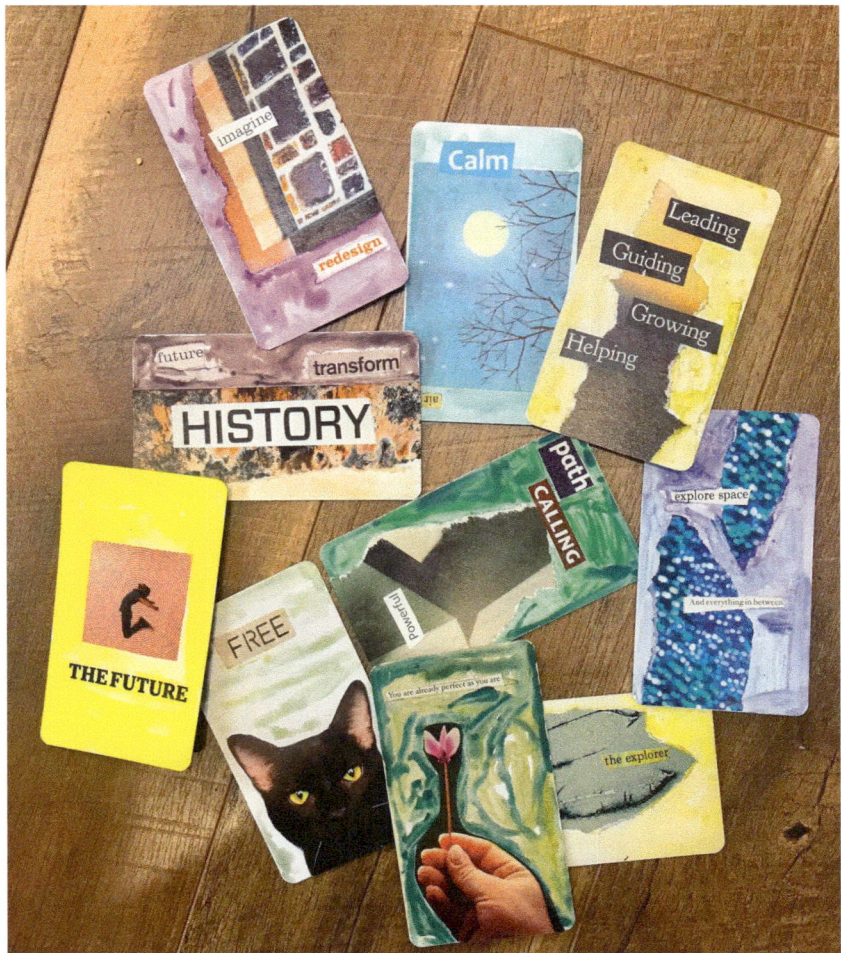

Figure 6.1 Mindfulness mantra cards.

Examples of phrases or words that could be added to cards:

- Emotion management: I forgive myself; breathe, let go of anger and see clearly; I listen lovingly to inner conflict and reflect until I find peace around it; I share my happiness with those around me.

- Ego building: I am in control; I trust myself; I am seen; I am beautiful; I know who I am and I am enough; I draw from my inner strength and light.
- Grief/loss: I am present in all that I do; I embrace the peace and quiet of the night; I feel the presence of those who aren't physically here.
- Addiction: Each step is taking me to where I want to be; I trust myself to make the best decisions: I trust my inner wisdom; I am present in all that I do.

Mandalas

Mandalas were created to represent the universe and originally came from China, Japan, and Tibet. Sand mandalas are still painstakingly created acknowledging the impermanence of life through a deeply reflective process. Mandala is the Sanskrit word for circle. They were first introduced into mental health by Carl Jung who not only used them with his clients but created mandalas himself. It was his opinion that not only did the Mandalas have a calming effect, but they also seemed to promote individuation and psychic integration (Henderson et al., 2007). In one study mandalas were used with college students and were found to decrease social anxiety (Bi & Yongfang, 2019) (Figure 6.2).

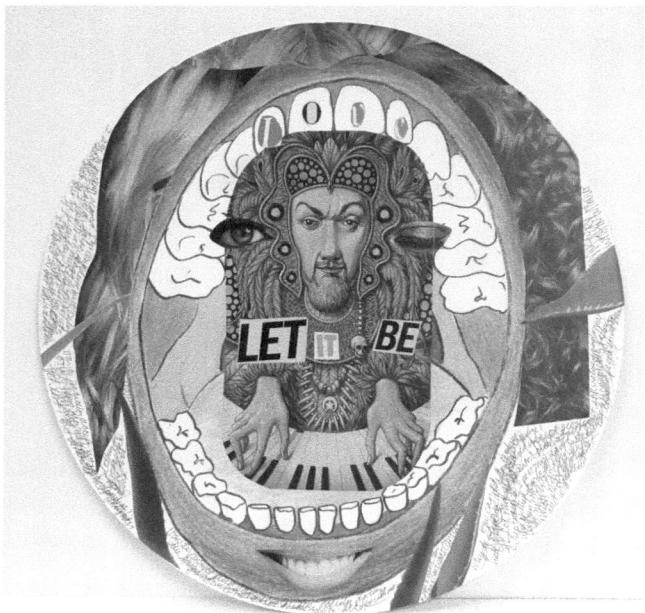

Figure 6.2 Mandala 1.

Art in circular form can be witnessed throughout the history of humankind. In Indigenous culture, a medicine wheel, dream catcher, or drum head could be considered a form of a mandala. In art history, a Grecian Labyrinth might be considered one, even Stonehenge could be considered a form of a mandala. Mandalas are also commonly used in art therapy practice with clients. Clinicians provide a pre-drawn circle and clients fill them in using various media. The circle can also represent a barrier or boundary in an art directive as seen in this section. When using the mandala as a prompt with clients it is important to honor the tradition of where the directive came from, appreciating the history and culture behind the practice and avoiding appropriation.

Rationale: Using the boundary of the circle the mandala can represent a safe space sometimes exploring what is on the outside. Performing a CMT meditation in relation to the prompt will further access unconscious material.

Inside/outside:

- Being alone/being with others
- What I can control/what I can't control
- Who is in my inner circle/who I keep outside: Focus on intimate and intentional relationships vs. shared history
- Honesty/dishonesty (Step 1 in the 12 steps of AA)
- Integrity/fragility (Step 5 in the 12 steps of AA)
- Humility/pride (Step 7 in the 12 steps of AA)

Materials: Paper with pre-drawn circles, pastels, markers, pencil, colored pencil, watercolor, collage.

The mandalas in Figure 6.3 were created by a cisgender adult female. She initially used oil pastels to create the image on the right and then laid paper over it and etched the design into the image on the left picking up the color from the oil pastels on the original drawing. The process was self-soothing to the client.

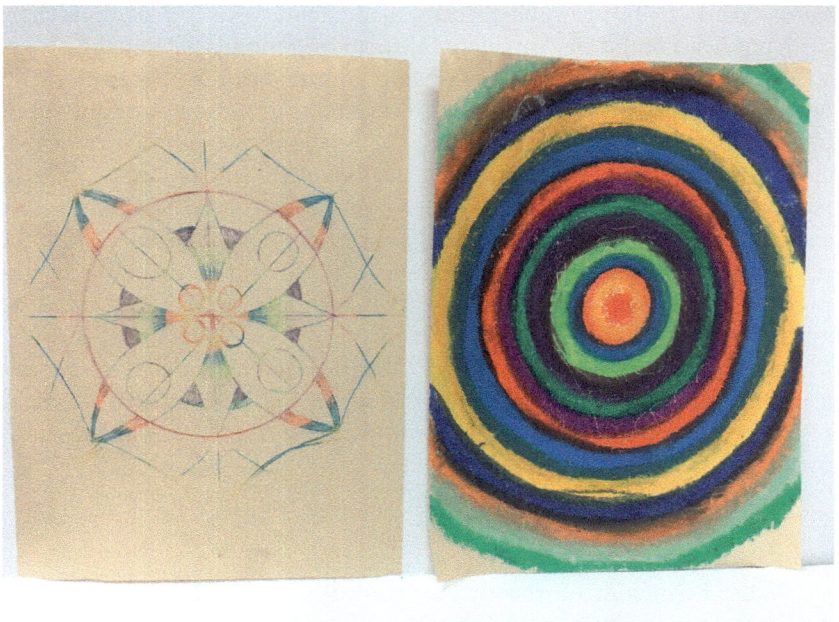

Figure 6.3 Mandala 2.

Tool Box

Rationale: This directive provides a tangible tool to utilize during a problematic emotional outburst. The box will hold contents that will be self-soothing resulting in increased self-regulation. Clinicians should begin with standard CMT protocol and then discuss the prompt to create the art piece. The client will decorate the outside of the box in session. The inside of the box will be a safe space also decorated by the client, but the client may also bring in personal items to add. Through the creation of this piece, clients will have the opportunity to explore and process beliefs and treatment targets. Additionally, clients will have a tool to assist in calming and relaxation skills outside of sessions. This directive is likely to take longer than one session. Figure 6.4 depicts the inside of a box created by a cisgender young adult female as a place to refer to when they needed to ground themselves.

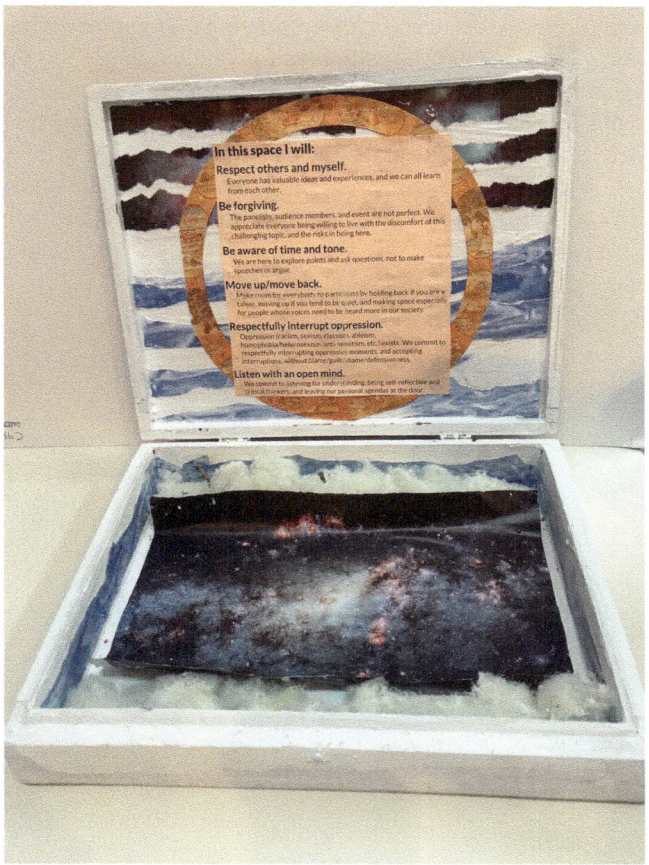

Figure 6.4 Tool box 1.

Prompts: Will vary depending on struggle/diagnosis and treatment planning.

- Grief: memory box which may include items honoring the loss (e.g. small item belonging to the deceased person, pictures, mementos/ ticket stubs from events)
- Anxiety: may include items that will help ground when intrusive thoughts come (e.g. stones, fabric pleasing to touch, comforting pictures)

Materials: Clients may use a wide variety of materials which may include paint, found objects, glitter, textured fabric, pre-cut collage images, glue, paintbrushes, hot glue, personal items the client adds.

Safe Space

Rationale: This directive provides clients an opportunity to explore what safe means to them. This directive is valuable for challenging thought distortions. The client will participate in a CMT guided meditation focusing on the concept of a safe space. The client should be instructed that the place they create might be a real place they have visited or a fantasy place they imagine. This directive will provide imagery that can be utilized in times when the client may be feeling triggered or out of control. Figure 6.5 depicts response art created by a cisgender young adult female.

   Art media: Pencils, pens, markers, paint, brushes, paper.

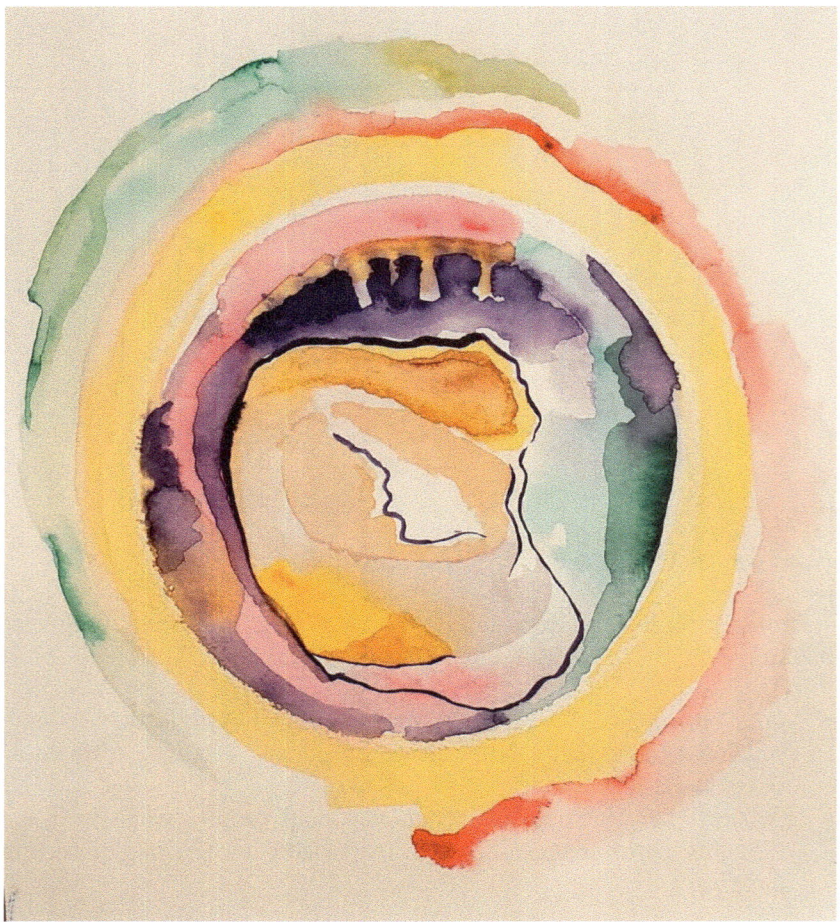

Figure 6.5 Safe space response art.

7 Self Reflection

This is me, I am...

Rationale: This directive will provide clients an opportunity to explore thoughts about themselves at the moment as well as their schema, the concept of self-talk, and beliefs. This directive will also aid in establishing rapport and building a therapeutic alliance. Clinicians should begin with standard CMT protocol suggesting the client meditate on the mantra *This is me, I am...* focusing on the current moment, not the past or the future. This directive and process will provide opportunities for clients to explore and challenge biases, distorted messages and work to build reality-based, positive, and realistic ideals that will boost their self-confidence when coping with unsound fears. If it is fitting, clients may explore active role transitions while engaging in this directive (e.g. achieving milestones, start or termination of a relationship or job, relocation). The verbal process could provide an opportunity to witness positive and difficult features as well as create opportunities for goal setting to attain proficiency in a new role. If the struggles relate to grief this directive provides a container for the narrative around the current circumstances of the loss, feelings, and the effects of loss. This directive is an informative assessment tool providing space for the characteristics of the struggle (e.g. type of loss/trauma, previous functioning vs. current functioning, coping mechanisms) and may be incorporated additionally towards the end of treatment to provide insights to growth by later comparing the two pieces. This directive will assist in assessing the client's self-perception and how the symptoms are exhibited within a clinical diagnosis (e.g. depression, social anxiety) to further direct treatment planning. Figure 7.1 is a mixed media collage illustrating the many facets of the self.

Art media: Pre-cut collage images, pencils, pens, markers, glue, scissors.

DOI: 10.4324/9781003036777-7

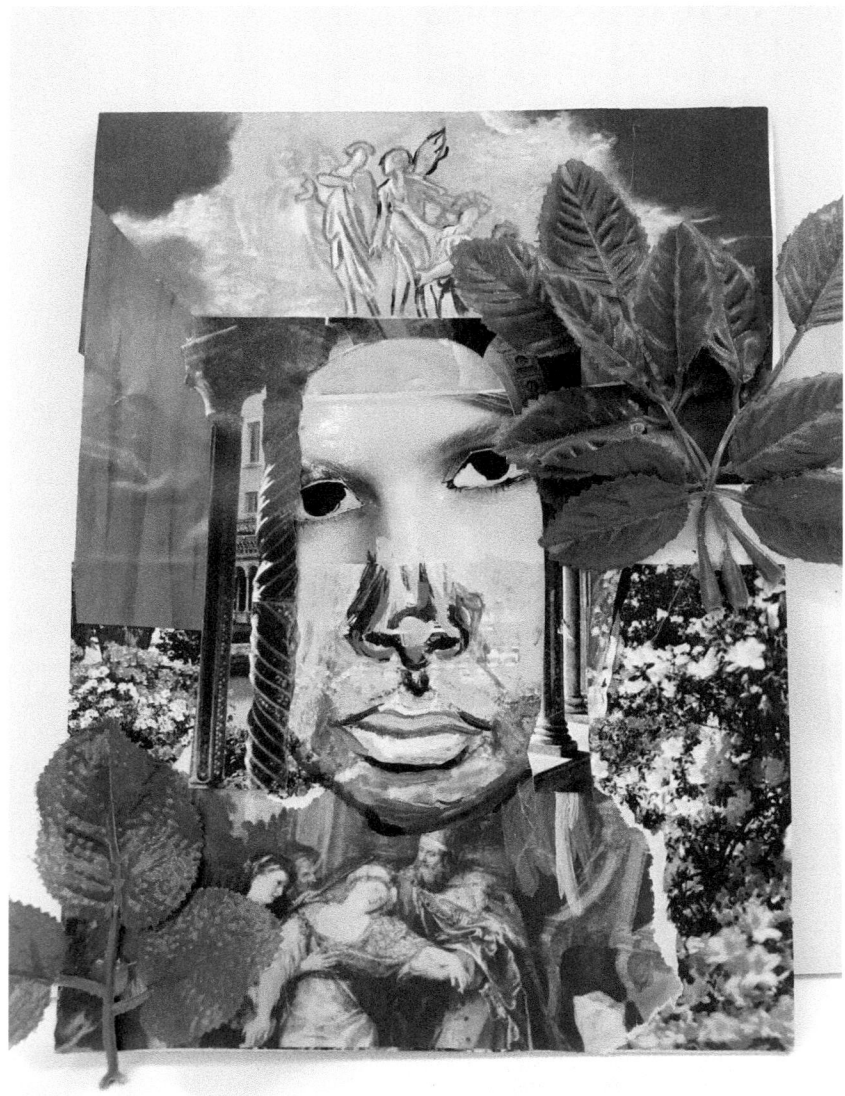

Figure 7.1 This is me I am... (1).

I come from...

Rationale: This directive provides clients an opportunity to explore thoughts about the past in a narrative piece. Themes that may be explored include unresolved life conflicts, which could lead to working on acceptance and resolution. Additionally, clients may explore beliefs about the self, including issues relating to safety, power, esteem, intimacy, trust, and control. Clinicians should begin with standard CMT protocol and then discuss the prompt to create the art piece. Prior to engaging in the art, the clinician should take a moment with the client to finish the sentence 2–3 times with the clinician modeling options that may be concrete (e.g. I come from Michigan, I come from home) and also some that are abstract (e.g. I come from laughter, I come from chaos). In the verbal process, the clinician should reinforce and support the client's process and insights around the impact of their past emotional pain or abuse (e.g. emotional, physical, and sexual) onto their present life experience. The process may also include assessment of any conflicts of age, gender, or cultures that may also inform described struggles offering further insights into the client's experience. If the client is in treatment for addiction this piece may provide insights on family history and life stresses that contribute to addiction. This directive is likely to require follow-up in the art journal. This directive will also aid in establishing rapport and building a therapeutic alliance. Due to the evocative nature of this directive, more controllable art mediums are suggested. Figure 7.2 was created by a nonbinary BIPOC individual in an individual telehealth session. After engaging in a mindfulness meditation they reported feeling their ancestors "in my bones." They also processed feelings relating to racial trauma and identity.

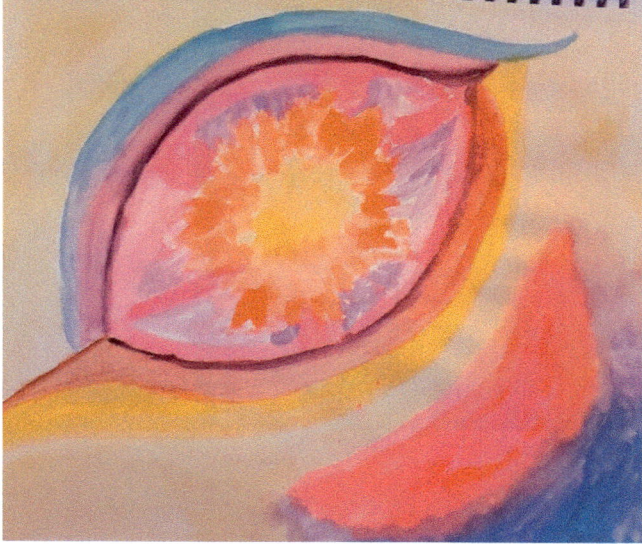

Figure 7.2 I come from....

Art media: Pre-cut collage images, pencils, pens, markers, glue, scissors, paper.

Beggar Bowl

Rationale: This directive is based on the concept of the Buddhist monks who use one bowl in many practical ways throughout their day (e.g. to collect resources, eating). Clinicians should begin with standard CMT protocol and then discuss the prompt to create the art piece. Afterward, the clinician should shift into a discussion about how needs and fulfillment feel in the body. Then the client will choose a vessel to embellish focusing on the outside of the vessel representing how they feel supported and the inside representing what they need to feel fulfilled. This piece is likely to take multiple sessions with CMT meditations focusing on the inside or the outside depending on where the client is in their process. This directive is designed to provide clients an opportunity to explore their needs. This directive and process will provide opportunities to assess and explore core conflicts from which their anxiety has manifested. Reflection on the outside will provide tangible insights to the client on meeting their needs. Figure 7.3 depicts a bowl created by a nonbinary adult individual. The strings represented boundaries.

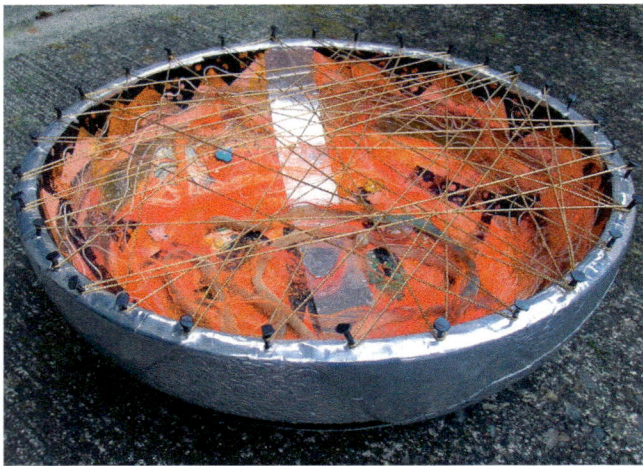

Figure 7.3 Beggar bowl.

Art media: Various vessels more specifically bowl-shaped and mixed media which may include paint, found objects, glitter, pre-cut collage images, glue, paintbrushes, hot glue. Clients may bring in personal items or images for this project.

What I Know for Sure

Rationale: This directive will provide clients an opportunity to explore and honor strengths in self and in life. This directive and process will provide opportunities for clients to explore unrealistic worries and biases, the concept of self-talk, and beliefs about the self. The clinician will guide the client in the CMT body scan from Chapter 5. Afterward, once the client is grounded the clinician will suggest a piece of art in response to the statement, "what I know for sure" assuring them there is not just one way to do this and to remember the process.

Art media: Pre-cut collage images, pencils, pens, markers, glue, scissors.

Inside/Outside Box

Rationale: This directive will provide the client with the opportunity to explore self-image. Clinicians should begin with standard CMT protocol and then discuss the prompt to create the art piece The outside of the box represents what the client shows the world, the inside of the box the intimate self that they only share with those they trust (refer to Chapter 2 Intimate Relationships in the 8 dimensions of wellness). Through the creation of this piece, clients will have the opportunity to explore and process self-concepts. This directive is likely to take longer than one session. Figure 7.4 depicts an inside/outside box created by a young adult cisgender BIPOC female using a wooden cigar box, hot glue, and paint. The outside appears dark and slightly intimidating while the inside vibrant with rich color and reflection protecting a fleshy heart.

Materials: Clients may use a wide variety of materials which may include paint, found objects, glitter, textured fabric, pre-cut collage images, glue, paintbrushes, hot glue, personal items the client adds.

I statements

Rationale: This directive provides opportunities for clients to self-perception and how one communicates their needs. This directive may also provide insights on expectations of others in relationships as well as assess if wants and needs are realistic and attainable. *I statements* may include:

* I feel...
* I want...
* I need...
* I am...

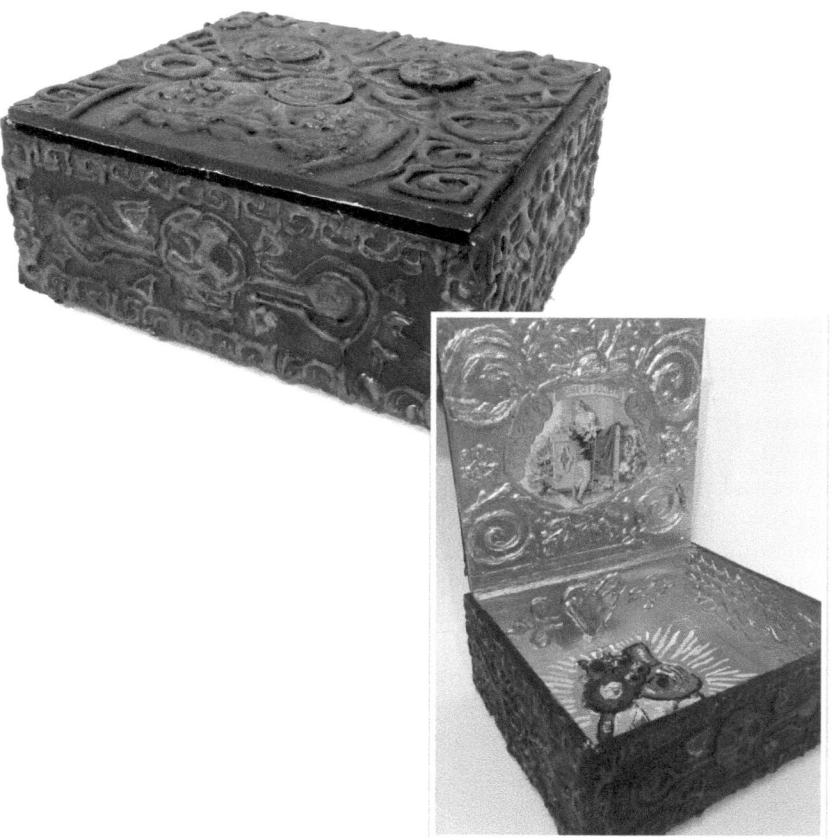

Figure 7.4 Box.

"I" statements are commonly used in therapy and are harmonious in the practice of mindfulness. They provide a tangible mantra to finish and can be very concrete (e.g. I feel hungry) or very abstract (e.g. I am running with the wolves). These sentences turned into art pieces provide effectual art pieces to reflect on outside of sessions. They can also be opportune art journal prompts. Clinicians should begin with standard CMT protocol and then discuss the prompt to create the art piece. Afterward, the client will engage in the art-making process in response to one of the statements. Choosing which statement can be up to the discretion of the clinician or the client depending upon the client's needs (both met and unmet) at the moment. Sometimes clients may avoid the "I" statement that might be the most fitting to explore in a session. This choice can be determined during the initial session check-in. Incorporating "I" statements in session check-ins adds to establishing structure in the therapeutic relationship, trust-building, and creating a safe environment for client disclosure. The ongoing practicing of the statements in session and in art journaling outside of sessions also aids in reducing anxiety around self-advocacy.

"I" statements lend themselves poignantly to some of the 12 steps in addiction work (e.g. I admit..., I believe..., I surrender..., I accept..., I am willing..., I forgive..., I can..., I commit...). Figure 7.5 depicts a mixed media piece of art created by a transgender nonbinary individual exploring the self.

Art media: Pre-cut collage images, pencils, pens, markers, glue, scissors.

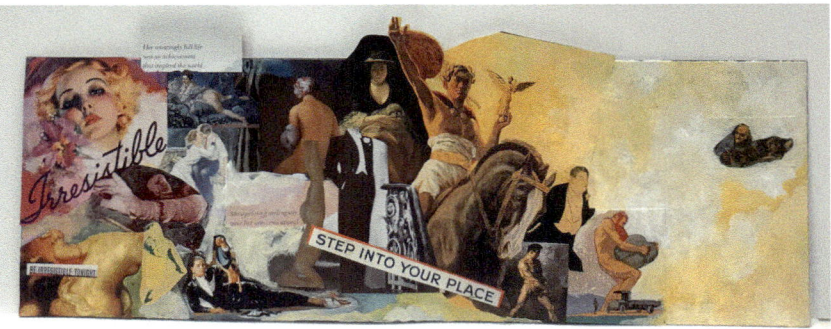

Figure 7.5 "I" statement game.

Tree

Rationale: This directive is informational when utilized early in treatment.

Clinicians should begin with standard CMT protocol, which may include imagery around trees. Afterward, the clinician will direct the client to consider how important trees are in humankind's existence. Trees provide the planet with oxygen and contribute to all living things. Trees also have to contend with struggles in their own survival. Trees sometimes become diseased. Trees also have to coexist with other creatures and humans, some helpful to the tree's existence and others damaging. After providing some of these thoughts to the client, the clinician will then suggest the client create a tree that represents them. The client should be sure to include space for the roots and what lies beneath the surface that is not seen. It does not matter if the tree is realistic or abstract as long as it represents them. The two pieces depicted in Figure 7.6 were created by the same cisgender young adult female. The tree on the left is from the first session and the tree on the right is from the final session. The client included words in the roots that she considered below the

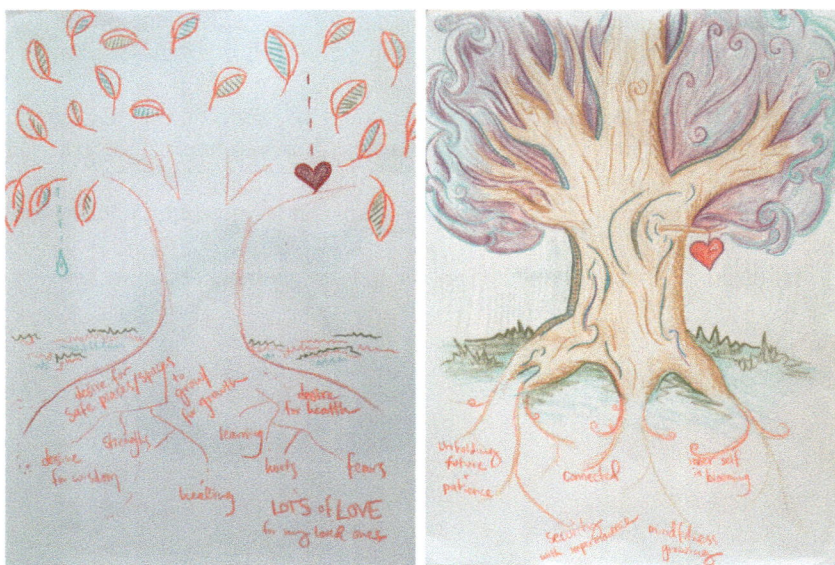

Figure 7.6 Trees.

surface and not accessible to all she encounters. In the first session, the client and clinician witnessed the piece and the client discussed some of the struggles that she saw in the tree. At times the client was tearful and observed a sort of transparency in the tree connecting it to feelings she had about herself. This client consistently attended 8 months of individual art therapy and over that span began to create art at home in her own time. The client became more independent, confident, and secure in her emotional wellness. In the final session, this client had not looked at the earlier piece that had been in storage but created a tree focused on how she was feeling about her life at that time. When the trees were compared the client acknowledged the growth she had experienced over the course of treatment.

Art media: Pre-cut collage images, tissue paper, colored paper, pencils, pens, markers, glue, scissors, paint.

8 Externalizing

Externalization is a defense mechanism providing an individual with a method of expression for a feeling or thought that may be conscious or unconscious. When one externalizes they project these feelings or thoughts into an action that may or may not be related to the origin resulting in a range of consequences depending on the act. When an individual is lacking in self-advocacy and constructive communication skills their outward reactions may include problematic behaviors (e.g. fighting, arguing, tantrums, stealing, lying, fire setting) (Helmond et al., 2015). Art therapy provides an alternate method for externalizing struggles resulting in feelings of control and opportunities for creative thinking. This provides a different perspective outside of the client's typical process. As the individual's outlook shifts, oftentimes deflating the severity of their feelings making them more manageable, the struggle transforms into a malleable piece of art. This process can also result in increased tolerance and resiliency over time. This chapter contains directives for individuals to specifically focus on the details of the conflict or the struggle outside of themselves providing a shift in perspective leading resulting in solutions and moving beyond problematic reactions (Ramey et al., 2009).

What does _____ look like?

Rationale: This directive provides clients an opportunity to see a specific struggle (e.g. anxiety, grief, trauma, depression, addiction) outside of them. This art directive also provides the opportunity to visually describe details of their history and externalize feelings. Clinicians should begin with standard CMT protocol and then discuss the prompt to create the art piece. The creation does not have to be realistic in depiction, an abstract shape may be easier to create for some clients. The client should be encouraged to imagine the entity with color, texture, or shape. The verbal process provides the opportunity for clients to dialogue with and explores how the struggle has impacted their daily functioning. It is also an opportunity to explore specifics including the excessiveness, frequency, intensity, and duration of symptoms as they occur. This process will also provide an opportunity to see how the body creates messages that may be helpful in identifying triggers. The clinician may

DOI: 10.4324/9781003036777-8

incorporate role-play in the verbal process, which may include role reversal with struggle. The clinician should be prepared to support the client with grounding techniques if triggered. This directive will also aid in establishing rapport and building a therapeutic alliance. Figure 8.1 depicts a mixed media collage by a nonbinary adult illustrating the externalization of anxiety around gender expression.

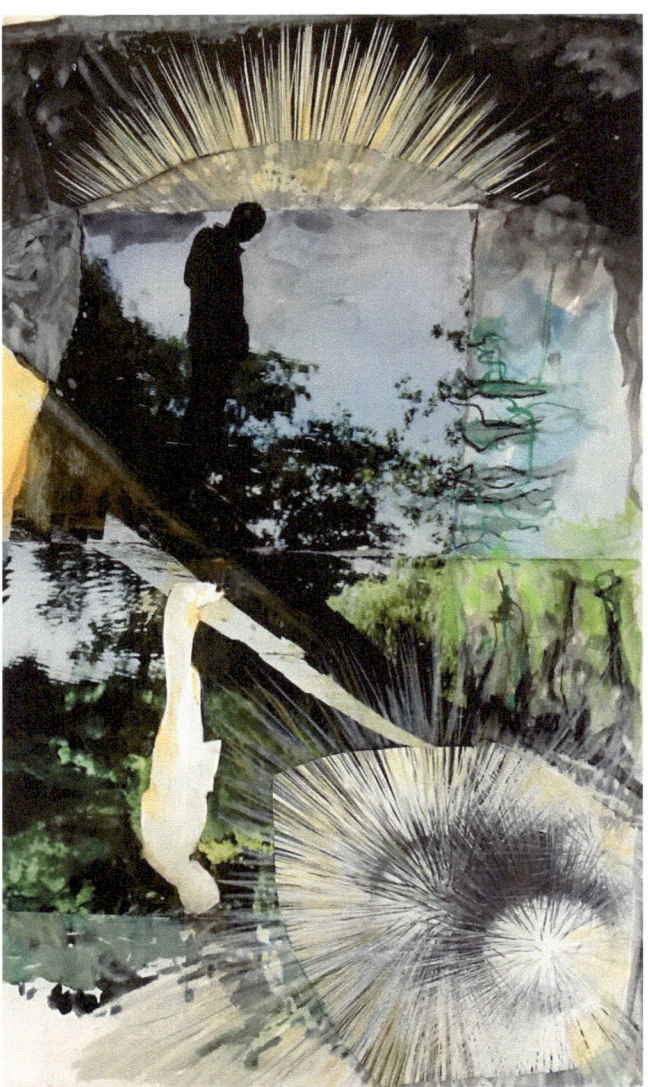

Figure 8.1 What does gender look like?

Art media: Colored paper, pencils, pens, markers, glue, scissors, paper.

Barometer

Rationale: Clinicians should begin with standard CMT protocol and then discuss the prompt to create the art piece. When the client is ready, the clinician will explore the idea of struggles (e.g. anxiety, grief, trauma, depression, addiction) having varying levels in relation to coping vs struggles and all the factors that are involved. This directive is intentionally called barometer, not thermometer, because a barometer can reflect more elements and circumstances that may provide opportunities for detailed life metaphors. A thermometer is more limited with just the choice of temperature. During the CMT guided meditation, the clinician could suggest the client imagine the barometer inside of their chest, the length of their spine. Afterward, the clinician will suggest the client create a barometer of their struggle considering temperature as well as external factors that may play into the experience. This directive provides clients an opportunity to see the varying experiences of their struggles and triggers. This directive also provides a scale of reference and self-assessment tool to utilize when experiencing triggers in daily functioning. This will also aid in developing a crisis plan if necessary. If the client is experiencing grief the stages of grief might be worked into the barometer providing options for education on the stages. Figure 8.2 was created by a gender queer BIPOC young adult and illustrates what the client created after guided imagery. The oval shape was described as a "seed" in their stomach and also related to traumatic emotional wounds they felt. During the creation of the response art, the client also created the spectrum barometer along the side depicting a range of feelings they regularly experienced in their body surrounding their eating disorder. The description of the range included the following details to connect with and check-in with both in and out of session connecting with the clinician for support when in crisis.

- Black: incapacitated
- Blue: depressed
- Red: feeling pain throughout the body and struggling with cognitive process
- Orange: pain in the stomach
- Yellow: a little anxiety
- Green: not feeling anxiety

The client struggled to describe green saying, "I don't know green very well." In this session, the client was able to discuss where and when to seek support. Support people were also identified.

Art media: Colored paper, pencils, pens, markers, glue, scissors, paper.

Struggle Container

Rationale: This directive provides a vessel to externalize unwarranted fears, anxiety, vulnerability, and other difficult feelings. The client will also have the

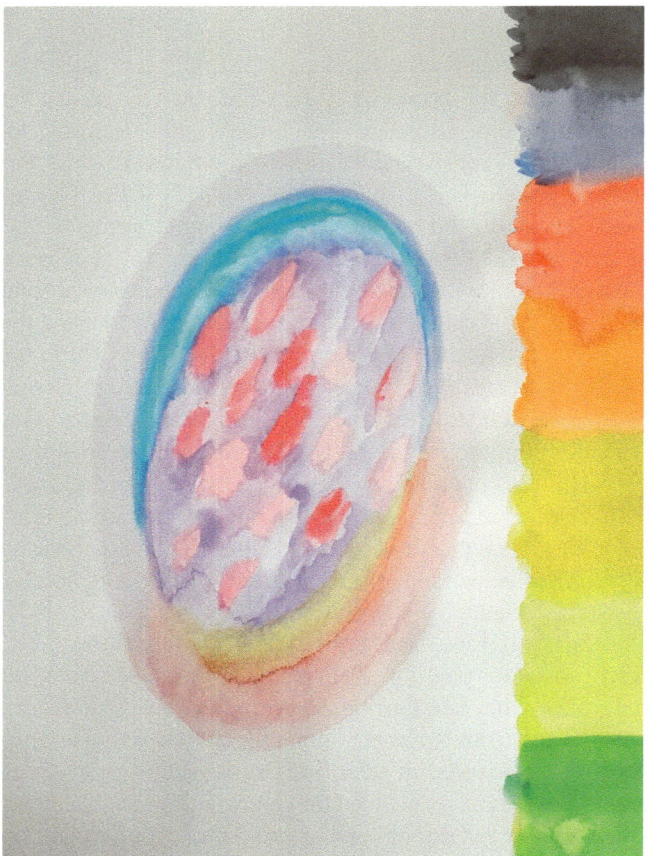

Figure 8.2 Barometer.

opportunity to explore beliefs through a verbal process. Clinicians should begin with standard CMT protocol and then discuss the prompt directions in creating the art piece. The meditation could focus on the idea of visualizing a container for the struggle (e.g. Anxiety, grief, trauma, depression, addiction). Over time outside of the session, the client may use the completed container as a place to write down and insert intrusive thoughts in daily life. The client can choose whether or not they want to be able to access the contents or have the container locked with an opening to insert these thoughts into. Container choices may vary from wooden cigar boxes, various bowls, bottles, or other vessels. It is best to have unique choices for the client to pick the right vessel. The clinician will suggest the client embellish the outside of the vessel in a way that the struggle is safely and securely held. This vessel may also be revisited later in treatment to reflect on and reinforce new thoughts and beliefs (may include power, control, safety, esteem, trust, and intimacy). Art journaling outside of the session may also be incorporated to explore and restructure underlying assumptions and beliefs that come up when adding to the container. Figure 8.3. depicts a struggle contained created by a queer adult female.

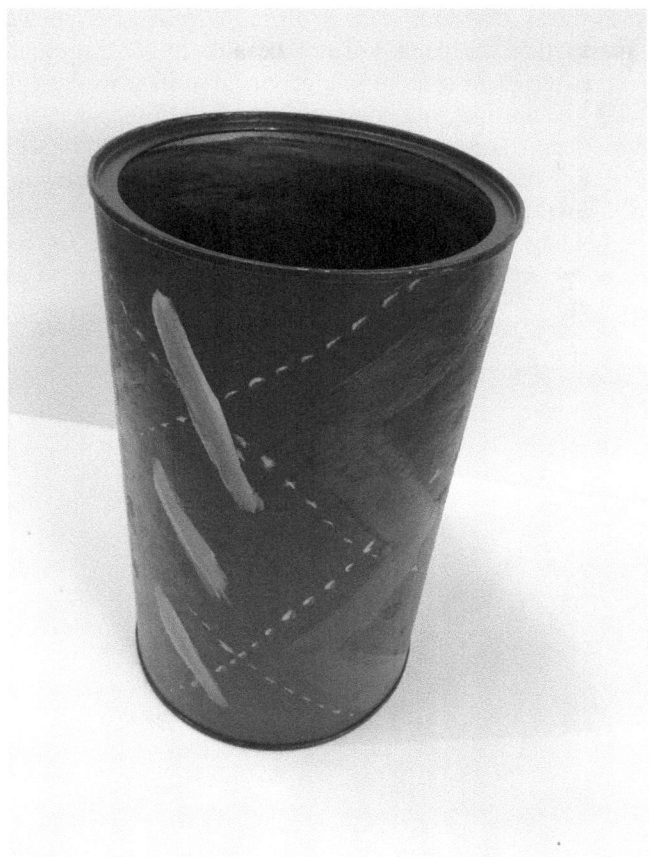

Figure 8.3 Struggle bottle.

Art media: Various vessels (boxes, bowls, bottles) to choose from and mixed media which may include paint, found objects, glitter, pre-cut collage images, glue, paintbrushes, hot glue.

It's OK

Rationale: This directive is designed to provide the client a place to forgive themselves. Clinicians should begin with the standard CMT protocol and then discuss the prompt directions in creating the art piece. The client will use a white crayon to free-write on the watercolor paper. Clients will work in a stream of consciousness approach writing statements around self-forgiveness.

The client will turn the paper one-quarter turn after filling it up eventually writing on the paper in each direction. The writing will not be able to be read. After they have finished writing the client will shift to watercolor paint and begin to add color any way that feels right to them. Wax resist from the writing will leave marks that the paint will not be able to soak through creating lines and curves the client can use to guide them in their work. The finished piece will likely be abstract, but some clients may find shapes in the process and develop them. The watercolor process after writing is self-soothing after externalizing often intense feelings. The white on white provides feelings of freedom to acknowledge and externalize the actions, feelings, and regrets they may be holding on to. This directive will provide space for re-solution and self-forgiveness. Figure 8.4 illustrates the wax resist process as described in the directive.

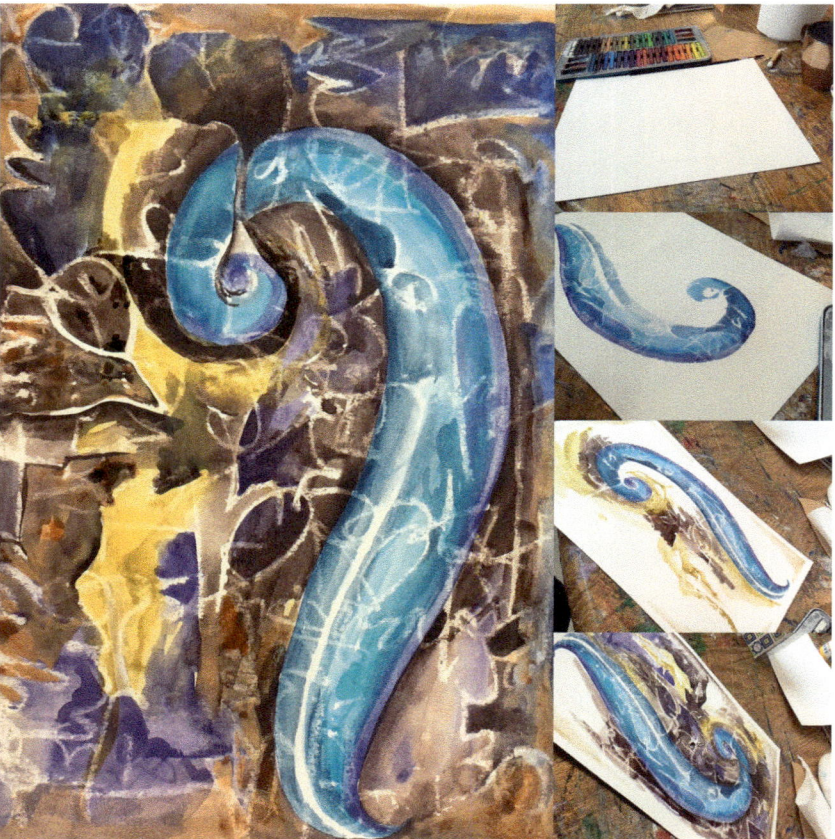

Figure 8.4 Wax resist process.

Art media: White crayon, watercolor paper, watercolor paint.

9   Working with It

Planting Seeds

Rationale: Clinicians should begin with standard CMT protocol and then discuss the prompt directions in creating the art piece. Guided imagery #4 in the Chapter may be utilized. Afterward, the clinician will suggest the client consider the idea of new growth and changes they would like to cultivate in their lives. These might include methods for coping, cognitive restructuring, or other life goals that address emergent struggles. They will then create a piece of art depicting seeds with flaps of paper that fold over the seeds they want to "plant" in their lives. This directive will provide opportunities to identify future situations to be "cultivated" or "weeded" as well as assist in goal setting. Art journals may be incorporated for tracking progress towards goals. The process may be ongoing as it is likely to include discussing relapses of symptoms or patterns. The process may also explore specifics around the implementation of goals. For clients in treatment for addiction multiple steps may be referenced in this directive (e.g. Step 10: discipline in maintaining sobriety, Step 11: cultivating awareness and spirituality, Step 12: acts of service). "Seeds" may assist the client in recognizing new opportunities for non-substance-related social experiences. This directive could also be applied in working with financial wellness for more concrete goals. Figures 9.1 and 9.2 (Short, 2016) depict the method of overlaying flaps in the mixed media art journal entry.

Art media: Pre-cut collage images, pencils, pens, markers, glue, scissors, paper, paint, brushes

My Struggle and My Relationships

Rationale: This directive provides clients an opportunity to explore beliefs about the self in relation to others including issues relating to safety, power, esteem, intimacy, trust, and control. Clinicians should begin with standard CMT protocol and then discuss the prompt directions in creating the art piece. The client will be directed to explore how their struggle (e.g. Anxiety, grief, trauma, depression, addiction) has impacted their relationships with

DOI: 10.4324/9781003036777-9

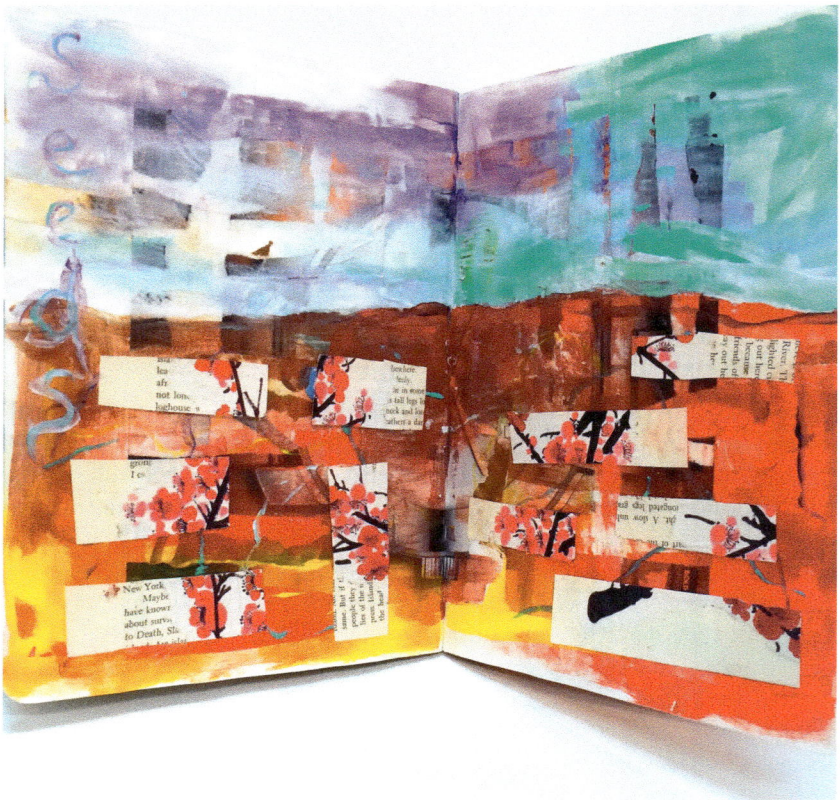

Figure 9.1 Planting seeds 1.

others. The clinician may refer to the five levels of social relationships of the 8 dimensions of wellness in Chapter 2. The process may include role-playing around communication with others. In the verbal process, this directive may also be helpful in understanding interpersonal disputes in past and current relationships, fears of rejection, past abandonment, and exploring and implementing conflict resolution skills (e.g. consistently communicating with respect, compromise, flexibility, listening when it is difficult, displaying appropriate levels assertiveness). In the session, the process may also address other interpersonal struggles. If relationships are at a standstill process may include the process around terminating a relationship if that is what is best for the client. Clinicians may utilize role-playing in session to dissipate feelings of anxiety around social interactions. Art journaling outside of sessions could be utilized to track struggles and success in relationships. If the client is struggling with grief, the process may include the person who passed. Grief work is likely to include addressing both social and emotional wellness (Chapter 4) working towards the expression and resolution of any

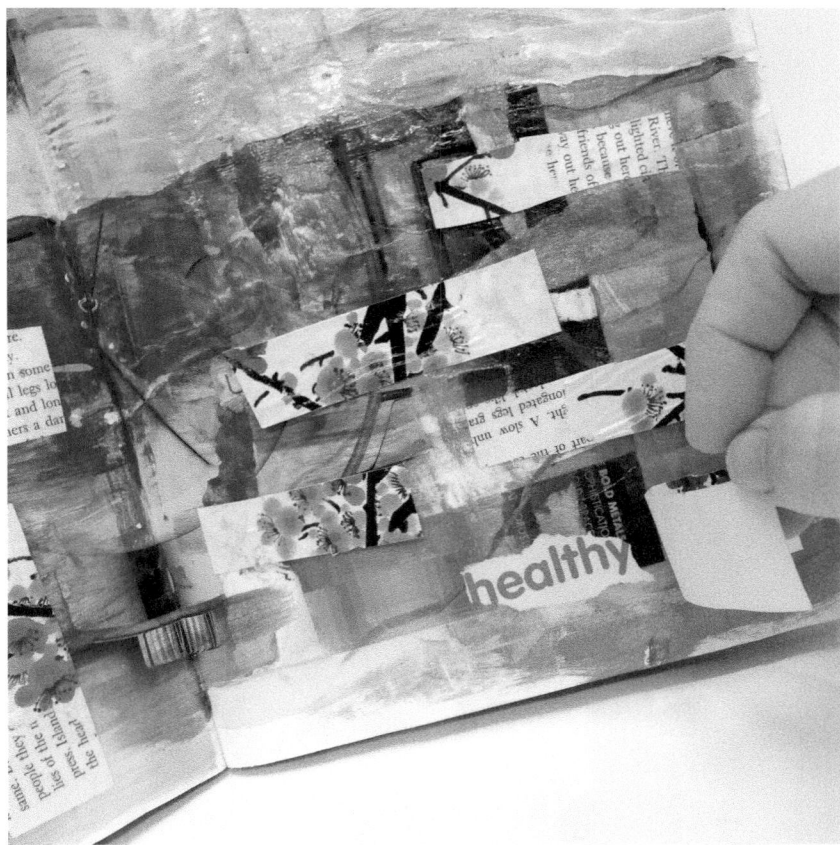

Figure 9.2 Planting seeds 2.

feelings of abandonment and the impact of the loss on other relationships. Work in an art journal outside of session may include exploring activities previously enjoyed and who was involved in them. For a client working with addiction, this directive could target Step 9 (making amends) of AA's 12 Steps. This may include verbal processes around the negative effects of substance abuse on family, friends, and vocational relationships and what amends may need to be made. The process may also include clinician engaging in role-playing with the client modeling communication skills that deliver an understanding of the consequences of their actions and an acceptance of responsibility for choices in efforts to solve the problem. Figure 9.3 was created by a nonbinary BIPOC individual in an individual telehealth session. In the figure, the session was near the winter holidays after a mindfulness meditation focus on life. Themes of the season included exploration around personal and professional relationships. Figure 9.4 was

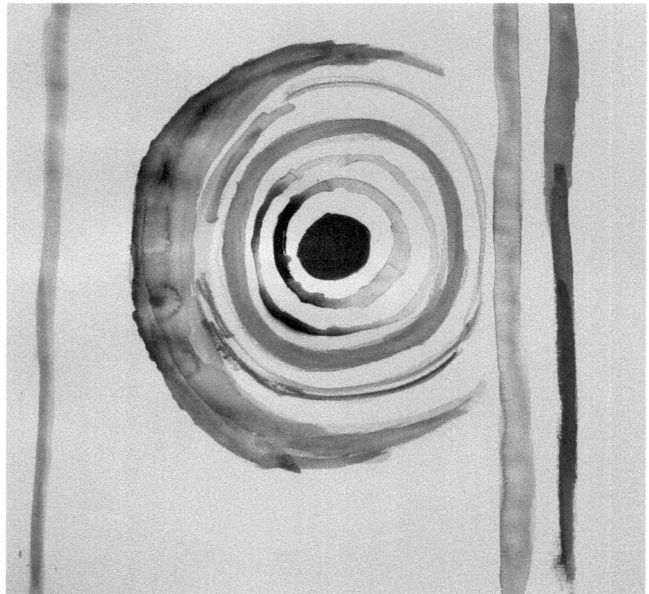

Figure 9.3 Response art: relationships.

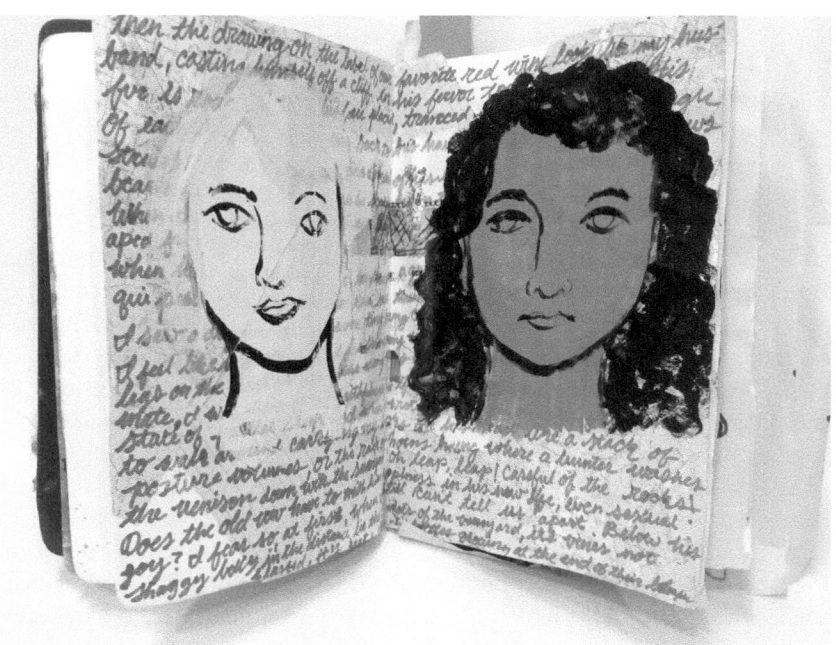

Figure 9.4 Relationships journal entry.

created by an adult cisgender female in a workshop focused on the social wellness aspects of the eight dimensions of wellness.

Art media: Pre-cut collage images, pencils, pens, markers, glue, scissors, paper.

My Struggle and My Environment

Rationale: This directive is designed to provide the client the opportunity to explore their home surroundings in relation to their environmental wellness. Clinicians should begin with standard CMT protocol with the focus being on imagining their home environment. Afterward, the client will create a piece of art exploring their home environment considering objects in the home that may create feelings of comfort and then also objects in the home that may bring up difficult feelings. Through the process, the client will consider items in the home that may be identified as triggers. Homework around this directive may include the client doing a walk-through and considering items that may need to be donated, or boxed up for storage to clear the trigger from their space. This directive would be helpful for those with hoarding tendencies. This art directive can be tailored to fit any of the formerly mentioned conflicts. Figure 9.5 was created by a cisgender young adult female using drawing materials

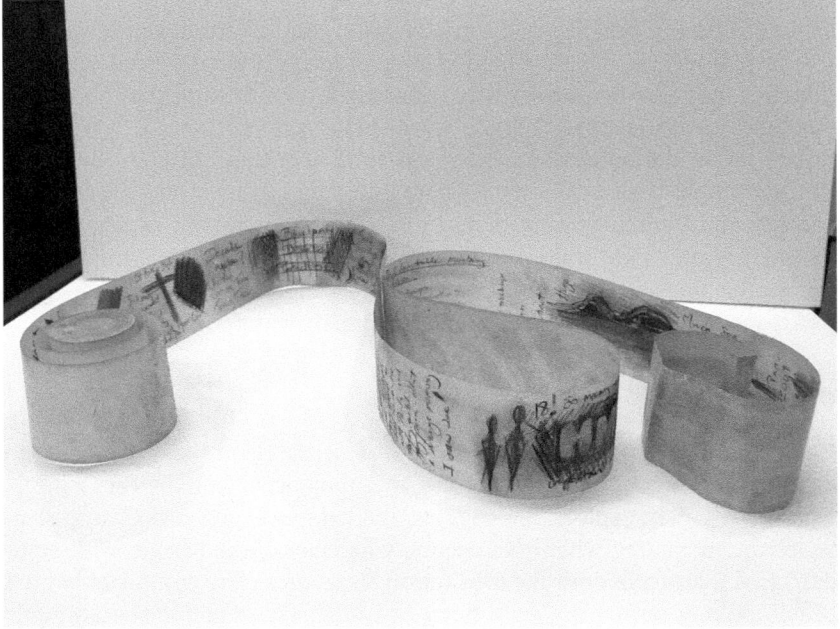

Figure 9.5 Response art: balancing the eight dimensions.

and tape from an adding machine turned into a scroll exploring life's journey.

Art media: Pencils, pens, markers, and paper.

Dear _____,

Rationale: This directive is designed especially for grieving to provide the client a place to say anything they were not able to say to a lost person. Clinicians should begin with the standard CMT protocol and then discuss the prompt directions in creating the art piece. Clients will use the white crayon to write a letter on the watercolor paper employing a wax resist technique. The client will turn the paper one-quarter turn after filling it up eventually writing on the paper in each direction. The writing will not be able to be read. After they have finished writing they will shift to watercolor paint and begin to add color any way that feels right to them. Wax resist from the writing will leave marks that the paint will not be able to soak through creating lines and curves the client can use to guide them in their work. The finished piece will likely be abstract, but some clients find shapes in the process and develop them. The watercolor process after writing is self-soothing after externalizing often intense feelings. The white on white provides feelings of freedom to acknowledge the actions, feelings, and regret they are holding on to. This directive will provide space for resolution and self-forgiveness. The verbal process may include a role-play with the piece/lost person responding to the letter. The process may include feelings around the last meaningful contact with that person, aspects or memories about the relationship, and exploration of supportive loved ones in life that could be included in the conversation. This directive may also be utilized with terminated relationships that hold grief and unresolved feelings. Figure 9.6 displays a piece created by a nonbinary adult individual. The letter was to their mother-in-law who chose to discontinue their relationship. The individual did not have any living parents and had cautiously begun to look at this person as a potential parental figure. This piece was processing the grief and confusion around the mother-in-law's response.

Art media: White crayon, watercolor paper, watercolor paint.

Relapse

Rationale: This directive is designed to provide the client the opportunity to explore moments of lapse and relapse that may occur in daily functioning. The process may explore the triggers, their impact, prevention, and strategies for managing when this occurs. Clinicians should begin with standard CMT protocol with the meditation focus on sitting comfortably on a beach looking out over a calm body of water. The clinician should guide the client to imagine what senses may be evoked sitting there. When the

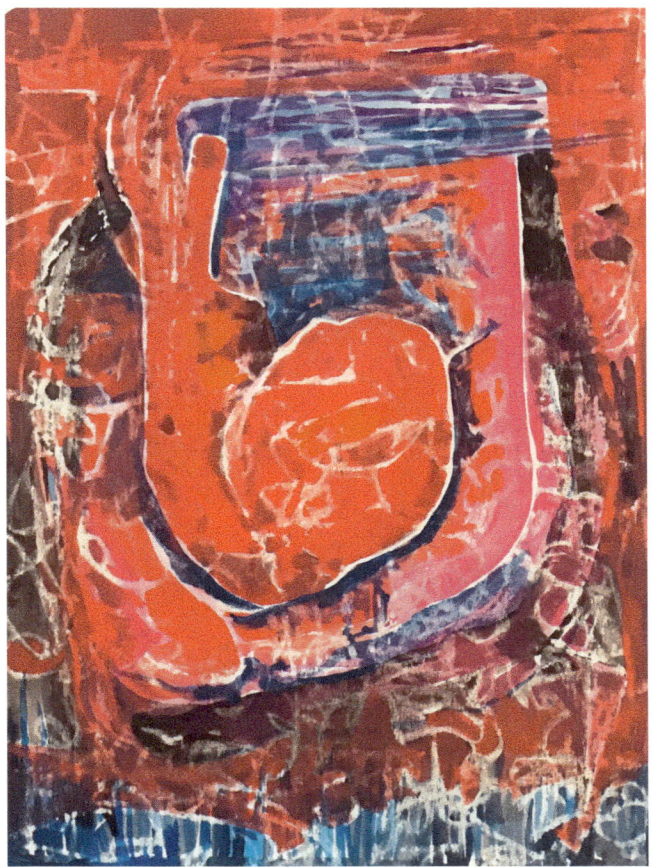

Figure 9.6 Open letter: wax resist.

session shifts to art-making the focus should be to create a piece of art depicting how the water changes when triggers come up in life. The process should include exploring behaviors, attitudes, feelings, and negative people or situations that may have impacted the relapse. Figure 9.7 illustrates an art journal entry created by a cisgender adult female depicting a multitude of feelings.

Art media: Pencils, pens, markers, oil pastels, and paper.

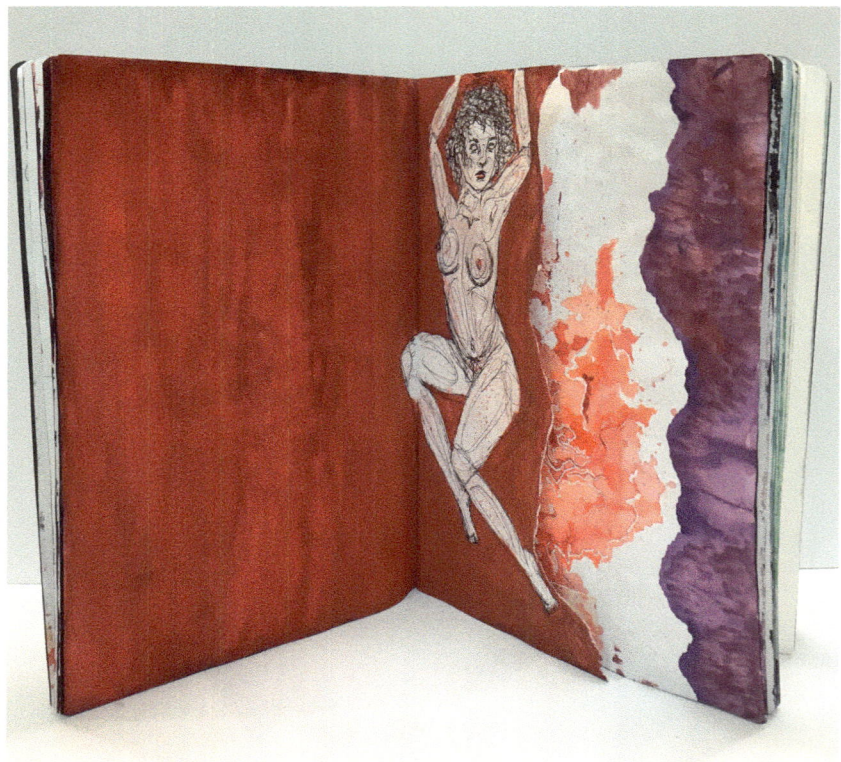

Figure 9.7 Relapse of emotion.

I Want You to Know

Rationale: This directive is designed to provide the client with a dialogue with their struggle (e.g. Anxiety, grief, trauma, depression, addiction). Clinicians should begin with the standard CMT protocol and then discuss the prompt directions in creating the art piece. The client will use a white crayon and the wax resist technique to free-write on the watercolor paper. The client will work in a stream of consciousness approach writing thoughts and feelings they want to say directly to their struggle. The client will turn the paper one-quarter turn after filling it up eventually writing on the paper in each direction. The writing will not be able to be read. After they have finished writing they will shift to watercolor paint and begin to add color any way that feels right to them. Wax resist from the writing will leave marks that the paint will not be able to soak through creating lines and curves the client can use to guide them in their work. The finished piece will likely be abstract, but some clients find shapes in the process and develop them. The watercolor process after writing is self-soothing after externalizing often intense feelings. The white on white provides feelings of freedom to externalize thoughts and feelings that may have felt scary to acknowledge. The verbal process should explore feelings, instead of avoiding or ignoring them. In the session, the process may also include role-play or verbal dialogue with the struggle (art piece).

Art media: White crayon, watercolor paper, watercolor paint.

10 Vicarious Trauma and the Clinician

Client work and trauma have been highlighted throughout this workbook, but it is imperative to also address the clinician's wellness. Working as a support person in mental health can be tremendously rewarding. It must also be stated that the role a clinician plays in the therapeutic alliance brings with it an enormous amount of responsibility. Clinicians hold a safe space for clients to explore and express an array of thoughts, patterns, and struggles in the work they do. Holding space requires dedication not only to the clients but also to their own wellness. The clinician's self-care requires taking into consideration all they absorb from sessions, seen, and heard. Incorporating consistent measures in self-care can alleviate the effects of this work diminishing the chances of early career burnout and vicarious traumatization.

The term vicarious trauma was created by McCann and Pearlman in 1990 and occurs when a clinician's ability to function both personally and professionally becomes at risk while providing treatment with clients of trauma (Way et al., 2007). Over time the client's experience of their trauma experience impacts the clinician's own "inner experience" (Pearlman & Saakvitne, 1995, p. 151). This can be magnified if the professionals have their own history of abuse or trauma. This tendency is not a surprise, as it is discussed throughout clinical training and often in continuing education, however, it is an ordeal that persists in this work. Vicarious trauma not addressed will eventually impact a clinician's ability to fulfill their job, this often leads to quicker turnover and high caseloads for those left doing the work. Vicarious trauma may also have a further impact on those working solely in private practice vs. those working on a team who have the support of others and consistent supervision (Harrison & Westwood, 2009).

The definition of vicarious trauma has evolved and can also occur through lived traumatic current events and struggles among others in the population. Social media makes headlines available moments after they occur and individuals often lack the boundaries to engage in shorter more manageable increments. In the year 2020, the collective trauma of humankind included personal losses due to the COVID-19 pandemic and a

DOI: 10.4324/9781003036777-10

divisive political climate in the United States. Wildfires spread in the United States and Australia resulting in many individuals losing their homes. The year 2020 also saw a collective of determined and resolved individuals challenging long-standing racism and white supremacy after shootings of BIPOC individuals became more forefront with accounts being contributed in real-time by witnesses to the crimes on to their individual social media lifting a veil of reality to many who had previously gone on oblivious to the unfair treatment of BIPOC individuals.

With social distancing, the new norm mental health professionals were forced to adapt by providing telehealth sessions to clients grappling with complex symptoms. While a limited number of clinicians had already begun this practice with contact restrictions, increased extreme personal losses, racism, and a contentious political climate the need for mental health treatment heightened. Clinicians adapted to support their clients with minimal in-person options, primarily in hospital settings. With the increase in telehealth also came an increase in options for online supervision, training, and consultation. This shift in service delivery brought work home where boundaries between work and personal life became less stringent and for many left self-care less of a priority.

In art therapy training, clinicians learn early on about *response art* (Moon, 1999). Response art provides a space for clinician self-reflection, as well as reflection in relation to a client and the art the client may have created (Fish, 2012, 2019; Drapeau et al., 2021). The process of making response art palliates the potential trauma experience (Gibson, 2018) and also provides space to illuminate the many inscrutable dynamics that may arise in regards to the client and treatment (Fish, 2012, 2019). Response art also activates concrete documentation of the process of witnessing another's experience (Drapeau et al., 2021) and may bring to the surface tensions that may have gone unnoticed in the unconscious (Fish, 2012). Akin to a client's process in art therapy, response art becomes a form of sublimation that may nurture taxed empathy (Fish, 2012, 2019) and has the potential to arouse self-awareness and growth in personal values, morals, and how one relates to another promoting acceptance and tolerance of all intersections that an individual may possess.

Methods of maintaining a consistent practice of making response art is personal to each clinician. A small sketchbook or art journal is accessible for quick response work between sessions and helpful when transitioning to the next client. Response art can be done alone or in a group setting. Many art therapists who provide group clinical supervision incorporate response art in sessions. Art therapy group supervision and consultation provide colleagues the opportunity to find empathy in their work and the collective experience decreases feelings of isolation, especially to those in private practice (Fish, 2012). Self-care should also incorporate other holistic practices that can be consistently maintained. Examining the eight dimensions of wellness may inform the individual of areas that are lacking structure and support, and provide more specific opportunities for strengthening boundaries and limits in specialized areas (Harrison & Westwood, 2009). Incorporating a consistent mindfulness and meditation practice in both personal and professional life also provides moments of clarity at times when one might be feeling overwhelmed. This chapter is a collection of process art created by clinicians either in response to clients or current events in the world. It is intended to encourage clinicians to incorporate process art into their own self-care and in supervision and consultation.

Figure 10.1 was created by a BIPOC art therapist after a mindfulness reflection focused on 2020. Upon reflection, they reported that many of the marks represented scribbles in the brain of events that are now memories. Upon reflection this individual voiced a desire to remember the beauty, people sharing, caring, and wanting to help strangers more than the dread. This individual also expressed feelings of empowerment from the marches and elevation of the "black and brown stories."

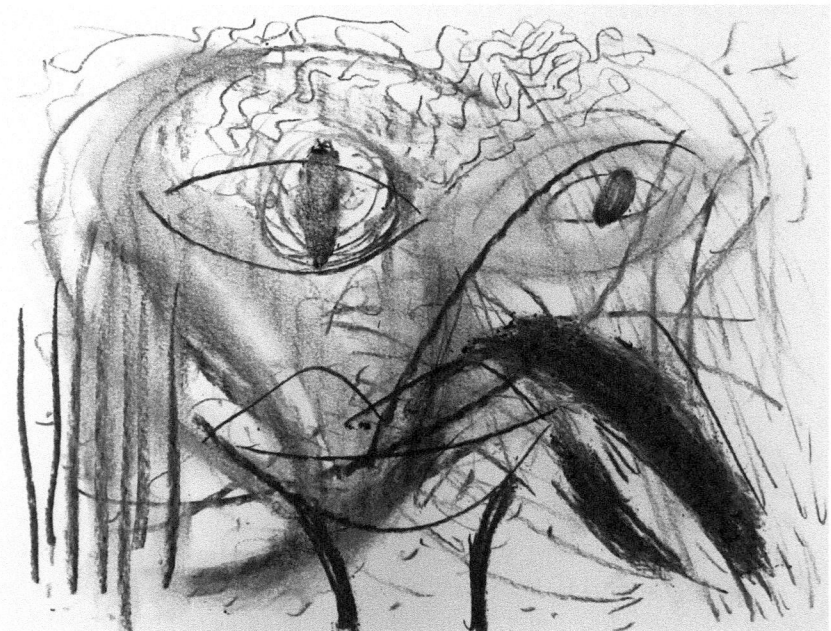

Figure 10.1 Clinician response art 1: 2020.

Figures 10.2−10.5 were created by a Latinx art therapist newly in the field. Figure 10.2 using black-out poetry was a response piece about an adult client who completed suicide. The client's daughter also had committed suicide prior.

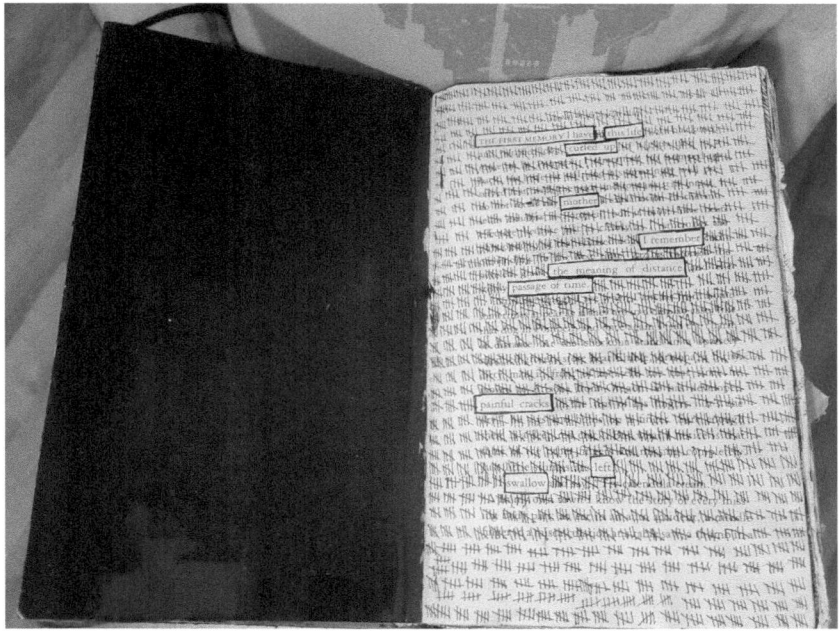

Figure 10.2 Clinician response art 1: suicide.

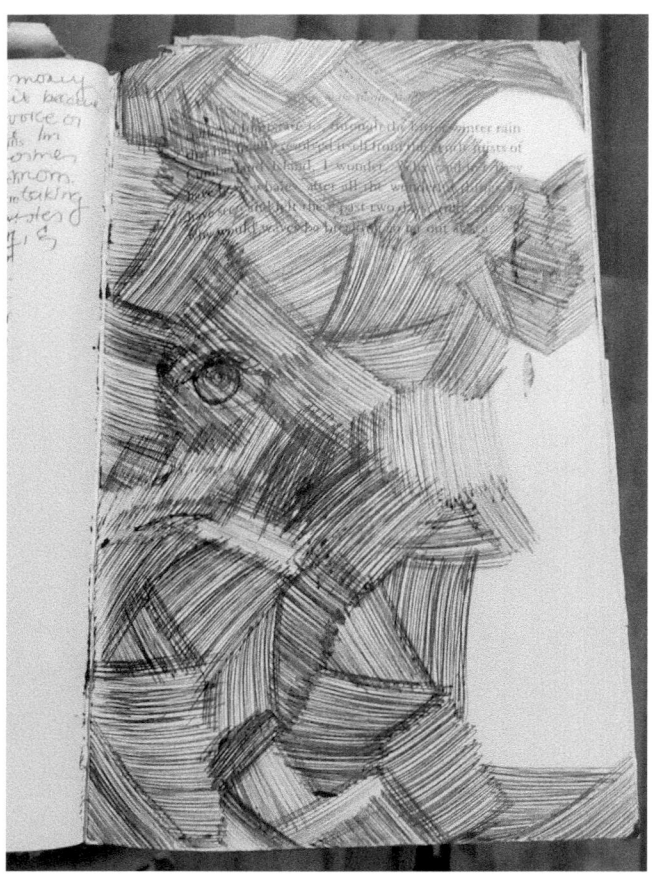

Figure 10.3 Clinician response art: soothing.

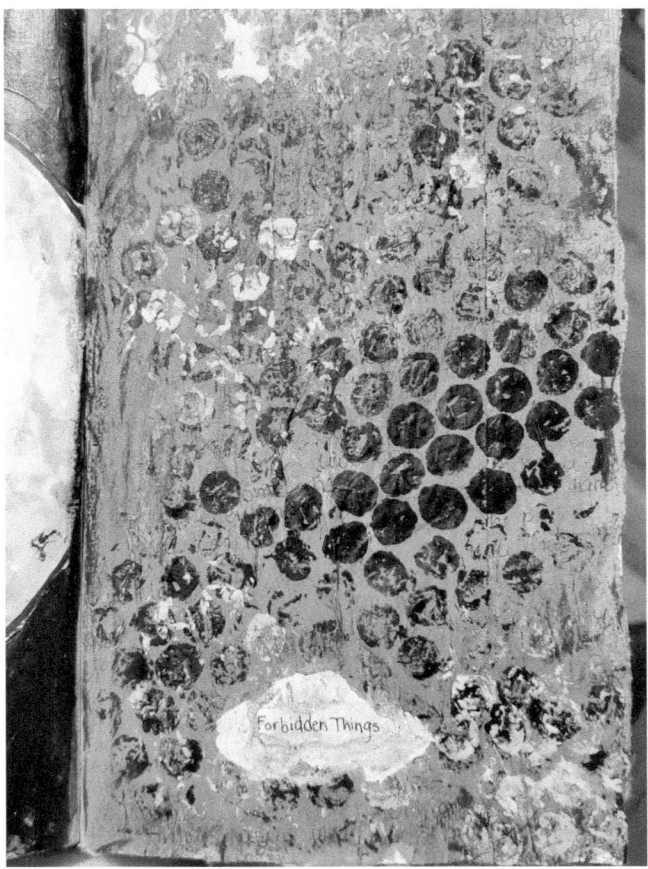

Figure 10.4 Clinician response art: transition into professional.

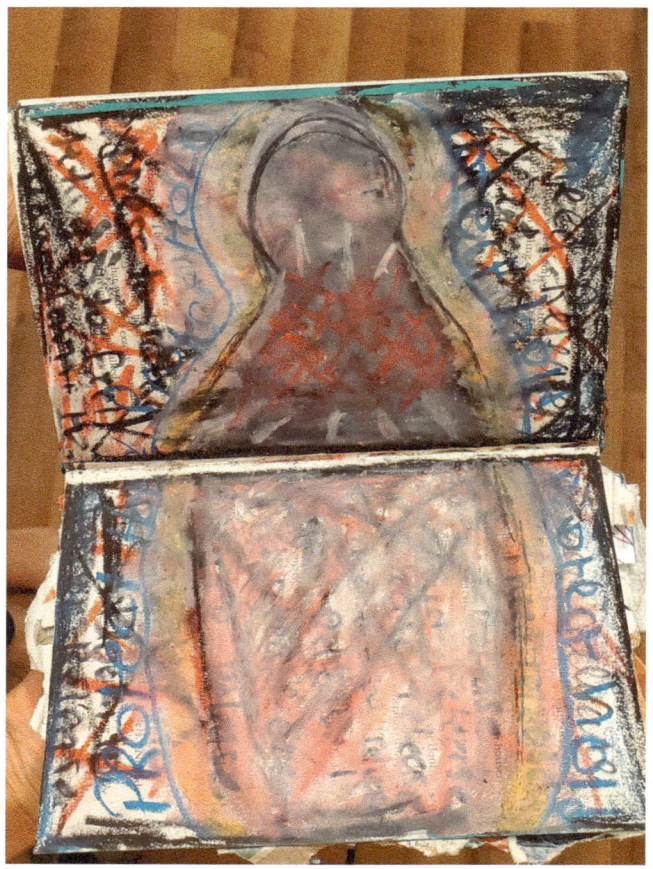

Figure 10.5 Clinician response art: rage.

Figure 10.3 was created as a self-soothing piece after sessions with clients.

Figure 10.4 was created when she was in the second year of school and in a new internship. This piece reflects feelings around working in mental health and imposter syndrome.

Figure 10.5 was created in the early days of the pandemic when the art therapist was in a training for a new job online that was hijacked and child pornography was played. The art therapist called this journal entry "Rage" and reported still having incredibly overwhelming anger many months later.

Figure 10.6 depicts an art therapist's process piece from group supervision. The clinician was processing navigating mental health systems.

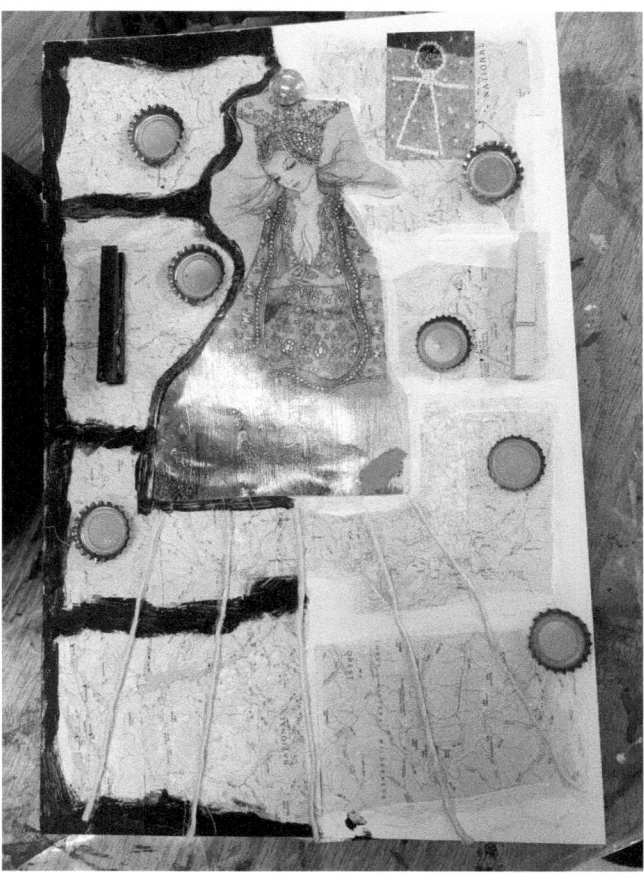

Figure 10.6 Clinician response art: navigating systems.

Figure 10.7 was created by an art therapist during an art therapy supervision group. This clinician was using the tree as a symbol of themselves both personally and professionally, balancing all facets of life.

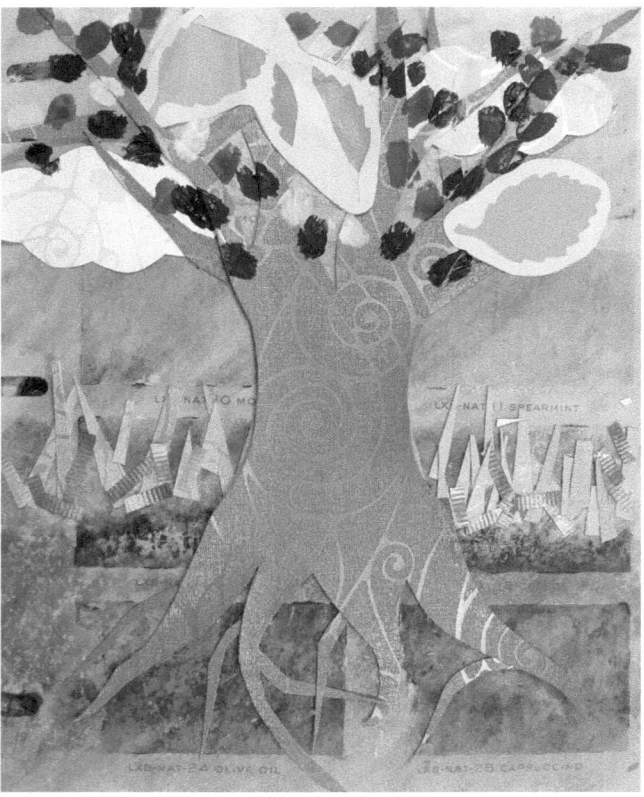

Figure 10.7 Clinician response art: tree.

Figure 10.8 depicts an art therapist's process art from an art therapy supervision group in response to creating a safe place for clients.

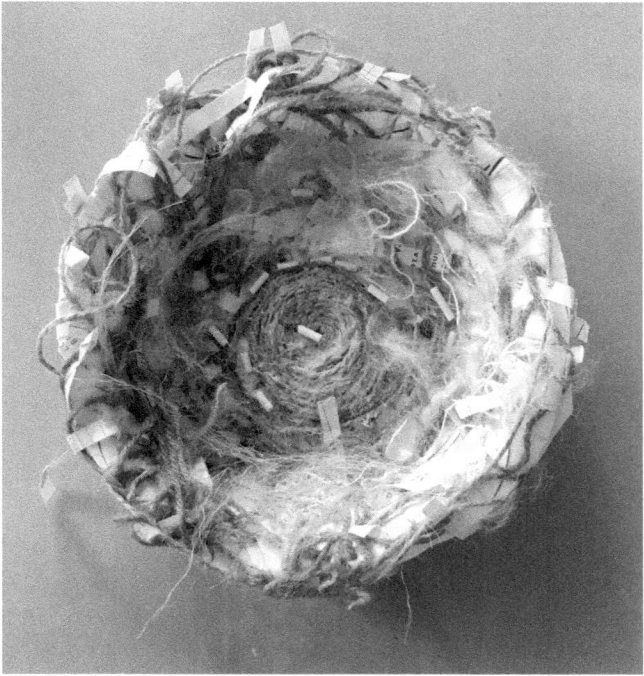

Figure 10.8 Clinician response art: nest.

References

Abbing, A., Ponstein, A., van Hooren, S., de Sonneville, L., Swaab, H., & Baars, E. (2018). The effectiveness of art therapy for anxiety in adults: A systematic review of randomised and non-randomised controlled trials. *Public Library of Science (PLoS) PLoS One, 13*(12), e0208716.

Agaibi, C.E., & Wilson, J.P. (2005). Trauma, PTSD, and resilience: A review of the literature. *Trauma Violence and Abuse, 6*(3), 195–216, https://doi.org/10.1177/1524 838005277438.

Alcoholics Anonymous World Services, Inc. (1989). *Twelve steps and twelve traditions.* Alcoholics Anonymous World Services.

Alzahrani, A.M., Hakami, A., AlHadi, A., Batais, M.A., Alrasheed, A., Abdullah, A., & Almigbal, T.H. (2020). The interplay between mindfulness, depression, stress and academic performance in medical students: A Saudi perspective. *Public Library of Science (PLoS) PLoS One, 15*(4), e0231088–e0231088.

American Art Therapy Association. (N.D.) *Art therapists training non-art therapists.* American Art Therapy Association. https://www.arttherapy.org/upload/ECTrainingNonATs.pdf.

American Psychiatric Association. (2013). *Diagnostic and statistical manual of mental disorders* (5th ed.).

Amutio, A., Franco, C., Pérez-Fuentes, M., Gázquez, J.J., & Mercader, I. (2014). Mindfulness training for reducing anger, anxiety, and depression in fibromyalgia patients. *Frontiers in Psychology, 5,* 1572. Frontiers Media S.A. https://doi.org/10.3389/fpsyg.2014.01572.

Art Therapy Credentials Board. (N.D.). *Code of ethics, conduct, and disciplinary procedures.* ATCB. https://www.atcb.org/Ethics/ATCBCode#1.5.

Avrahami D. (2006). Visual art therapy's unique contribution in the treatment of post-traumatic stress disorders. *Journal of Trauma & Dissociation, 6*(4), 5–38,

Berg-Cross, L., Craig, K., & Wessel, T. (2001). Multiculturalism at historically black colleges and universities: A case study of Howard University. In J. G. Ponterotto, J. M. Casas, L. A. Suzuki, & C. M. Alexander (Eds.), *Handbook of multicultural counseling* (2nd ed., pp. 849–870). Sage.

Bill, W. (1939). *Alcoholics anonymous: The big book.* Ixia Press, an imprint of Dover Publications, Inc. 2019.

Bi, Y., & Yongfang, L. (2019). Creating mandalas reduces social anxiety in college students. *Social behavior and personality, 47*(10), 1–10. Scientific Journal Publishers, Ltd.

Cardinal, R. (1972). *Outsider art*. Praeger Publishers.

Clark, C., Classen, C.C., Fourt, A., & Shetty, M. (2014). *Treating the trauma survivor: An essential guide to trauma-informed care*. Taylor & Francis Group.

Costello, C. (2015). *Developing resiliency practices in master's level counseling students through creative mindfulness training: An exploratory study*. ProQuest Dissertations Publishing.

Costello, C. (2021). *Creative mindfulness techniques for clinical trauma work*. Taylor and Francis.

Cronkleton, E. (2019). *Breathwork basics, uses, and types*. Healthline. https://www.healthline.com/health/breathwork#uses

Csikszentmihalyi, M. (1990). *Flow: The psychology of optimal experience*. Harper Collins.

Csikszentmihalyi, M. (1996). *Creativity: Flow and the psychology of discovery and invention*. Harper Collins.

Davidson, R.J., & Kaszniak, A.W. (2015). Conceptual and methodological issues in research on mindfulness and meditation. *The American Psychologist, 70*(7), 581–592. American Psychological Association.

Drake, J. E., Coleman, K., & Winner, E. (2011). Short-term mood repair through art: Effects of medium and strategy. *Art Therapy, 28*(1), 26–30. Taylor & Francis Group.

Drapeau, C.E., Drouin, M., & Plante, P. (2021). Vicarious trauma and response art: A professional development workshop for psychotherapists working with survivors of trauma. *The Arts in Psychotherapy, 72*, 101744.

Feng-Ying, H., Hsu, A., Hsu, L., Tsai, J., Huang, C., Chao, Y., Hwang, T., & Wu, C.W. (2019). Mindfulness improves emotion regulation and executive control on bereaved individuals: An fMRI study. *Frontiers in Human Neuroscience, 12*, 541. Frontiers Media S.A.

Fish, B.J. (2012). Response art: The art of the art therapist. *Art Therapy, 29*(3), 138–143. Routledge.

Fish, B.J. (2019). Response art in art therapy: Historical and contemporary overview. *Art Therapy, 36*(3), 122–132. Routledge.

Franklin, M. (2016).Contemplative wisdom traditions in art therapy. In J. Rubin (Ed.), *Approaches to art therapy: Theory and technique* (3rd ed., pp. 308–329). Routledge: Taylor and Francis.

Fraumeni-McBride, J. (2019). Addiction and mindfulness; Pornography addiction and mindfulness-based therapy ACT. *Sexual Addiction & Compulsivity, 26*(1–2), 42–53. Routledge.

Gerge, A., & Pedersen, I.N. (2017). Analyzing pictorial artifacts from psychotherapy and art therapy when overcoming stress and trauma. *The Arts in Psychotherapy, 54*, 56–68. Elsevier Ltd.

Gibson, D. (2018). A visual conversation with trauma: Visual journaling in art therapy to combat vicarious trauma. *Art Therapy, 35*(2), 99–103. Routledge.

Gidney, C., (2015). Nutritional wastelands: Vending machines, fast food outlets, and the fight over junk food in Canadian school. *Canadian Society for the History of Medicine, 32*(2), 391–409. Canada: Canadian Society for the History of Medicine.

Grof, S., & Grof, C. (2010). *Holotropic breathwork: A new approach to self-exploration and therapy*. State University of New York Press.

Halsey, B. (1977). Freud on the nature of art. *American Journal of Art Therapy*, *16*, 99–103.

Hampson, M., Ruiz, S., & Ushiba, J. (2020). Neurofeedback. *NeuroImage*, *218*, 116473. Elsevier Inc.

Hanes, M.J. (2007). "Face-to-face" with addiction: The spontaneous production of self-portraits in art therapy. *Art Therapy*, *24*(1), 33. Routledge.

Harrison, R.L., & Westwood, M.J. (2009). Preventing vicarious traumatization of mental health therapists: Identifying protective practices. *Psychotherapy Research Practice Training*, *46*(2), 203–219. Psychotherapy.

Hartz, L., & Thick, L. (2005). Art therapy strategies to raise self-esteem in female juvenile offenders: A comparison of art psychotherapy and art as therapy approaches. *Art Therapy*, *22*(2), 70. Routledge.

Helmond, P., Overbeek, G., Brugman, D., & Gibbs, J.C. (2015). A meta-analysis on cognitive distortions and externalizing problem behavior: Associations, moderator, and treatment effectiveness. *Criminal Justice and Behavior*, *42*(3), 245–262.

Henderson, P., Rosen, D., & Mascaro, N. (2007). Empirical study on the healing nature of mandalas. *Psychology of Aesthetics, Creativity, and the Arts*, *1*(3), 148–154. American Psychological Association.

Herman, J. (1992). *Trauma and recovery*. Basic Books.

Hinz, L.D. (2015). Media considerations in art therapy: Directions for future research. In D. E. Gussak & M. L. Rosal (Eds.), *The Wiley handbook of art therapy* (pp. 135–145). John Wiley & Sons.

Hinz, L.D. (2017). The ethics of art therapy: Promoting creativity as a force for positive change. *Art Therapy*, *34*(3), 142–145. Routledge.

Hinz, L.D. (2020) *Expressive therapies continuum: A framework for using art in therapy*. Routledge.

Jain, F.A., Connolly, C.G., Moore, L.C., Leuchter A.F., Abrams, M., Ben-Yelles, R.W., Chang, S.E., Ramirez Gomez, L.A., Huey, N., Lavretsky, H., & Iacoboni, M. (2019). Grief, mindfulness and neural predictors of improvement in family dementia caregivers. *Frontiers in human neuroscience*, 13. Frontiers Media S.A.

Jongsma, Arthur E., Jr., Peterson, L.M., & Bruce, T.J. (2014). *The complete adult psychotherapy treatment planner: Includes DSM-5 updates*. John Wiley & Sons, Incorporated.

Kabat-Zinn, J. (1990). *Full catastrophe living: Using the wisdom of your body and mind to face stress, pain, and illness*. Doubleday Dell Publishing Group.

Kabat-Zinn, J. (1994). *Wherever you go, there you are: Mindfulness meditation in everyday life*. Hyperion.

Kapitan, L. (2015). Social action in practice: Shifting the ethno-centric lens in cross-cultural art therapy encounters. *Art Therapy*, *32*(3), 104–111. Routledge.

Karcher, O. (2017). Sociopolitical oppression, trauma, and healing: Moving toward a social justice art therapy framework. *Art Therapy*, *34*(3), 123–128. Routledge. https://doi.org/10.1080/07421656.2017.1358024

Kendi, I.X. (2019). *How to be an antiracist*. One World.

Kramer, E. (1972). *Art as therapy with children*. Schocken Books.

Kramer, E. (1979). *Childhood and dart therapy*. Schocken Books.

Kramer, E. (2016). Sublimation in art therapy. In J. Rubin (Ed.), *Approaches to art therapy: Theory and technique* (3rd ed., pp. 71–87). Routledge.

Kübler-Ross, E. (1970). *On death and dying*. Routledge.

Kwan, L.Y., Leung, A.K., & Liou, S. (2018). Culture, creativity, and innovation. *Journal of Cross-cultural Psychology*, *49*(2), 165–170. Sage.

Leclerc, J., & Drapeau, C.E. (2018). Response art as reflective inquiry: Fostering awareness of racism. *The Arts in Psychology*, *60*, 9–18. Elsevier.

Lusebrink, V.B. (1990). *Imagery and visual expression in therapy*. Plenum Press.

Lusebrink, V.B. (2004). Art therapy and the brain: An attempt to understand the underlying process of expression in art therapy. *Art Therapy: Journal of the American Art Therapy Association*, *21*(3), 125–135. Routledge.

Lusebrink, V.B. (2010). Assessment and therapeutic application of the expressive therapies continuum: Implications for brain structures and functions. *Art Therapy*, *27*(4), 168–177. Routledge.

Malchiodi, C.A. (2012a). Art therapy and the brain. In C. A. Malchiodi (Ed.), *Handbook of art therapy* (2nd ed., pp. 17–26). The Guilford Press.

Malchiodi, C.A. (2012b). Expressive arts therapy and multimodal approaches. In C. A. Malchiodi (Ed.), *Handbook of art therapy* (2nd ed., pp. 130–140). The Guilford Press.

Malnutrition in America. (2019). Focus for health. https://www.focusforhealth.org/malnutrition/

Manteau-Rao, M. (2016). *Caring for a loved one with dementia: A mindfulness-based guide for reducing stress and making the best of your journey together*. New Harbinger Publications.

Mauss, I.B., Bunge, S.A., & Gross, J.J. (2008). Culture and automatic emotion regulation. In M. Vandekerckhove, C. von Scheve, S. Ismer, S. Jung, & S. Kronast (Eds.), *Regulating emotions: Culture, social necessity, and biological inheritance*. Blackwell Publishing Ltd.

McGoldrick, M., & Hardy, K.Y. (2008). Introduction: Re-visioning family therapy from a multicultural perspective. In M. McGoldrick & K. V. Hardy (Eds.), *Re-visioning family therapy: Race, culture, and gender in clinical practice* (pp. 3–24). The Guilford Press.

Moon, B.L. (1999). The tears make me paint: The role of responsive artmaking in adolescent art therapy. *Art Therapy: Journal of the American Art Therapy Association*, *16*(2), 78–82.

Pascual-Leone, A., Gillespie, N.M., Orr, E.S., & Harrington, S.J. (2016). Measuring subtypes of emotion regulation: From broad behavioural skills to idiosyncratic meaning-making. *Clinical Psychology and Psychotherapy*, *23*(3), 203–216. Wiley Subscription Services, Inc.

Pearlman, L.A., & Saakvitne, K.W. (1995). *Trauma and the therapist: Counter-transference and vicarious traumatization in psychotherapy with incest survivors*. Norton.

Pénzes, I., van Hooren, S., Dokter, D., Smeijsters, H., & Hutschemaekers, G. (2014). Material interaction in art therapy assessment. *The Arts in Psychotherapy*, *41*(5), 484–492.

Ramey, H.L., Tarulli, D., Frijters, J.C., & Fisher, L. (2009). A sequential analysis of externalizing in narrative therapy with children. *Contemporary Family Therapy*, *31*(4), 262–279.

Randal, C., Pratt, D., & Bucci, S. (2015). Mindfulness and self-esteem: A systematic review. *Mindfulness*, *6*(6), 1366–1378. Springer US.

Rasmussen, M.K., & Pidgeon, A.M. (2011). The direct and indirect benefits of dispositional mindfulness on self-esteem and social anxiety. *Anxiety, Stress, and Coping, 24*(2), 227–233. Taylor & Francis Group.

Robbins, A. (1998). *Therapeutic presence: Bridging expression and form*. J. Kingsley.

Robbins, A. (2012). Psychoanalytic, analytic, and object relations approaches. In C. A. Malchiodi (Ed.), *Handbook of art therapy* (2nd ed., pp. 57–74). The Guilford Press.

Robbins, A. (2016). Object relations and art therapy. In J. Rubin (Ed.), *Approaches to art therapy: Theory and technique* (3rd ed., pp. 126–138). Routledge.

Rubin, J. (2003). *The role of creativity in art therapy and art education. Canadian Art Therapy Association Journal, 16*(1), 10–16.

Rubin, J. (2016). Discovery and insight in art therapy. In J. Rubin (Ed.), *Approaches to art therapy: Theory and technique* (3rd ed., pp. 71–87). Routledge.

Sackett, C.R., & McKeeman, A. (2017). Using visual journaling in individual counseling: A case example. *Journal of creativity in mental health, 12*(2), 242–248. Routledge.

Sandmire, D.A., Gorham, S.R., Rankin, N.E., & Grimm, D.R. (2012). The influence of art making on anxiety: A pilot study. *Art Therapy, 29*(2), 68–73.

Saul, J. (2014). *Collective trauma, collective healing: Promoting community resilience in the aftermath of disaster*. Routledge.

Schmanke, L., (2015). Art therapy and substance abuse. In D. E. Gussak & M. L. Rosal (Eds.), *The Wiley handbook of art therapy* (pp. 361–374). John Wiley & Sons.

Scotland-Coogan, D. & Davis, E. (2016). Relaxation techniques for trauma. *Journal of Evidence-Informed Social Work, 13*(5), 434–441. Routledge.

Shore, A. (2006). Some personal and clinical thoughts about trauma, art, and world events. In F. Kaplan (Ed.), *Art Therapy and Social Action: Treating the World's Wounds* (pp. 175–190). Jessica Kingsley Publishers.

Shore, A. (2014). Art therapy, attachment, and the divided brain. *Art Therapy, 31*(2), 91–94. Routledge.

Short, B.A. (2016). *Creative wellness: Art journaling with mindfulness*. Violet Rose Publishing House.

Short, B.A. (n.d.). Artist/humankind: Location/earth. Retrieved January 1, 2021, from http://bethannshort.com/ahle.html

Siegel, D.J. (2010). *Mindsight: The new science of personal transformation*. Bantam Books.

Snir, S., & Regev, D. (2013). A dialog with five art materials: Creators share their art making experiences. *The Arts in Psychotherapy, 40*(1), 94–100. Elsevier Ltd.

Springham, N. (2008). Through the eyes of the law: What is it about art that can harm people? *International Journal of Art Therapy, 13*(2), 65–73. https://doi.org/10.1080/17454830802489141

Springham, N., & Huet, V. (2018). Art as relational encounter: An ostensive communication theory of art therapy. *Art Therapy: Journal of the American Art Therapy Association, 35*(1), 4.

Stoler, D.R. (2014, October 17). Neurofeedback: How does it work? *Psychology Today*. https://www.psychologytoday.com/us/blog/the-resilient-brain/201410/neurofeedback-how-does-it-work.

Strohmaier, S., Jones, F.W., & Cane, J.E. (2021). Effects of length of mindfulness practice on mindfulness, depression, anxiety, and stress: A randomized controlled experiment. *Mindfulness, 12*(1), 198–214. Springer Nature B.V.

Sue, D.W., Bernier, J.E., Durran, A., Feinberg, L., Pederson, P.B., Smith, E.J. & Vasquez-Nuttal, E. (1982). Position paper: Cross-cultural counseling competencies. *The Counseling Psychologist*, 10, 45–52. Sage.

Sue, D.W., & Sue, D. (2008). *Counseling the culturally diverse: Theory and practice* (5th ed.). John Wiley & Sons.

Swan-Foster, N. (2016). Jungian art therapy. In J. Rubin (Ed.), *Approaches to art therapy: Theory and technique* (3rd ed., pp. 71–87). Routledge.

Talwar, S. (2010). An intersectional framework for race, class, gender, and sexuality in art therapy. *Journal of the American Art Therapy Association, 27*(1), 11–17. Routledge.

Talwar, S. (2015). Culture, diversity, and identity: From margins to center. *Art Therapy, 32*(3), 100–103. Routledge.

Tang, Y., Hölzel, B.K., & Posner, M.I. (2015). The neuroscience of mindfulness meditation. *Neuroscience, 16*(4), 213–225. Springer Science and Business Media LLC.

Ter Maat, M.B. (2011). Developing and assessing multicultural competence with a focus on culture and ethnicity. *Journal of the American Art Therapy Association, 28*(1), 4–10. Taylor and Francis Group.

Thompson, B.L., & Waltz, J.A. (2008). Mindfulness, self-esteem, and unconditional self-acceptance. *Journal of Rational-Emotive and Cognitive-Behavior Therapy, 26*(2), 119–126. Springer US.

Thornton-Dill, B., & Zambrana, R.E. (2009). Critical thinking about inequality: An emerging lens. In B. Thornton-Dill & R. E. Zambrana (Eds.), *Emerging intersections: Race, class, and gender in theory, policy, and practice* (pp. 1–21). Rutgers University Press.

van der Kolk, B. (2014). *The body keeps the score: Brain, mind, and body in the healing of trauma*. Penguin Books.

Way, I., VanDeusen, K., & Cottrell, T. (2007). Vicarious trauma: Predictors of clinicians' disrupted cognitions about self-esteem and self intimacy. *Journal of Child Sexual Abuse, 16*(4), 81–98. Taylor & Francis Group.

Wilson, M. (2012). Art therapy in addictions treatment: Creativity and shame reduction. In C. A. Malchiodi (Ed.), *Handbook of art therapy* (2nd ed., pp. 302–319). The Guilford Press.

Wise, S. (2015). On considering the role of art therapy in treating depression. In D. E. Gussak & M. L. Rosal (Eds.), *The Wiley handbook of art therapy* (pp. 350–360). John Wiley & Sons.

Zeki, S. (2001). Artistic Creativity and the Brain. *Science, 293*(5527), 51. https://link.gale.com/apps/doc/A76697748/AONE?u=lacc_legal&sid=AONE&xid=6bcd3850

Index

ability/disability 21
addiction 19, 45–46, 48, 50–51, 79,
        81–82, 85–86, 92
ADHD 35
age 5, 73
Alcoholics Anonymous World
        Services, Inc., 1989 52
altered books 16–17
American Art Therapy Association
        (AATA) 2
American Psychiatric Association 39
Amutio, A. 42–43
anger 36, 42–43, 66, 100
anxiety 12, 32–33, 35, 41–42, 48, 50–51,
        69, 74, 77, 79–82, 85–86, 92
art, process of 9
art directives 20–21
Artist/Humankind: Location/ Earth
        (AH:LE) 9
art journaling: eight dimensions of
        wellness 48; feeling check in 49;
        gratitude 48; ritual 51–52; self-
        talk 50–51; strengths 52;
        supporting *The 12 Steps* 52–54;
        worry to relaxation 51–52;
        See also externalizing
art journals 47
art mediums 14–20
art mediums, properties of:
        controllable vs. fluid 15;
        indelible vs. easy to change 15;
        linework vs. swaths of color 16;
        simple vs. complex 15; small vs.
        large motor activity 16; soft vs.
        saturated color 16; structured
        vs. unstructured 15–16
art therapy, and PTSD 39–41

Art Therapy Credentials Board
        (ATCB) 2
art therapy directive 13
attachment 11–13
autism 35

barometer 81
beggar bowl 74–75
be here now 24–25
"black and brown stories" 96
Black Lives Matter 29
body scan 55–58
books, art mediums 16–17
bowls and other vessels, art
        mediums 17
boxes, art mediums 17
breathwork 36

Cardinal, Roger 9
Caregiver Summit 10
childhood trauma 40
Child Nutrition Programs 32
children, grief in 43–44
citizenship 5
class 6
clay, art mediums 17–18
clinician, vicarious trauma and 94–103
CMT *See* Creative Mindfulness
        Technique (CMT)
CMT applications: addiction 45–46;
        anxiety 41–42; depressive
        disorders 42–43; grief 43–44;
        low self-esteem 44–45;
        PTSD 39–41
codes of conduct 29
cognitive/symbolic level, ETC 14
collage, art mediums 18

collective tramua 21
control 72
Costello, Corrina 1
COVID-19 pandemic 26–28, 94–95
creative level, ETC 14
creative mindfulness mantra
     cards 64–66
Creative Mindfulness Technique
     (CMT) 1, 21, 25, 39; formal
     steps of CMT 34–35
Creative Mindfulness Techniques for
     Clinical Trauma Work 1
Csikszentmihaly, M. 24–25

Davidson, R.J. 24
Dear_____ 90
Dementia 44
depression 33, 35, 45, 48, 50–51, 69, 79,
     81–82, 85–86, 92
depressive disorders 42–43
diet and nutrition 32
digital media, art mediums 18
doll and puppet making, art
     mediums 18
drawing materials, art mediums 18
DSM-V 42
dynamically oriented art therapy 23

Eight Dimensions of Wellness:
     emotional wellness 25–26;
     environmental wellness 30–31;
     financial wellness 33;
     intellectual wellness 29–30;
     occupational wellness 33;
     physical wellness 31–33; social
     wellness 26–28; spiritual
     wellness 28–29
eight dimensions of wellness 48
emotional wellness 25–26
energy ball, variation of 59–60
esteem 72
ethnic background 25
ethnicity 6
Expressive Therapies Continuum
     (ETC) 4, 13–14
externalizing: barometer 81; it's OK
     83–84; struggle container
     81–83; what does _____
     look like? 79–80

failure, feelings of 32
family culture 25
feeling check in 49

fiber, art mediums 18
financial/socioeconomic status 5
financial wellness 33
flow state 24
found objects, art mediums 18
Freud, Sigmund 23

gender 6, 21, 25, 29, 73, 80
gender expression 5
Gender Summit 10–11
generalized anxiety disorder
     (GAD) 41–42
Gerge, A. 39
glass, art mediums 18–19
gratitude 48–49
Grecian Labyrinth 67
grief 26, 36, 42–45, 48, 50–51, 79,
     81–82, 85–86, 90, 92
grief/loss 66, 79
grief work 86–87
Grof, Christina 36
Grof, Stan 36
guided imagery: example 1 body scan
     55–58; example 2 variation on
     an energy ball 59–60; example 3
     safe place in nature 60–62;
     example 4 inner plant 62–63

Hanes, M.J. 46
headachess 35
Herman, J. 40
Hinz, L.D. 4
Huet, V. 12
hypervigilance 41

I come from 72–74
"inner experience" 94
inner plant 62–63
inside/outside box 75
intellectual wellness 29–30
intentional relationships 27
"intersectional scholarship" 5
intimacy 72
I statements 75–77
it's OK 83–84
I want you to know 92–93

Jongsma, Arthur E. 41
Jung, Carl 23

Kabat-Zinn, Jon 1, 24
Kagin, Sandra 14–20
Karcher, O. 5, 21
Kaszniak, A.W. 24

Kendi, Ibram X. 29
kinesthetic/sensory level, ETC 14
Kramer, Edith 23
Kübler-Ross, Elisabeth 43

life conflicts 72
low self-esteem 44–45
Lusebrink, Vija 14–20

mandalas 66–68
masks and body casting, art
        mediums 19
material experience 21
material interaction 21
McCann, I.L. 94
meditation 24
meditative art 36
memory 35
metal embossing, art mediums 19
micronutrient-realted malnutrition 32
migraines 35
mindfulness 1
mindfulness, alternative supports used:
        breathwork 36;
        neurofeedback 35–36
mindfulness, eight dimensions of
        wellness 42
Mindfulness-Based Stress Reduction
        (MBSR) 24
Mindfulness-Based Stress Reduction
        (MBSR) program 1
mindfulness mediation 24
mixed media 20
mood repair 47
Moon, Bruce 34
multicultural competence 5
multicultural considerations 21–22
my struggle and my
        environment 89–90
my struggle and my
        relationships 85–89

nature, safe place in 60–62
Naumberg, Margaret 23
neurofeedback 35–36
nutritional wastelands 32

occupational wellness 33
outsider artists 9

painting materials, art mediums 19
panic attacks 35

Pearlman, Laurie 94
Pedersen, I.N. 39
perceptual/affective level, ETC 14
performance art, art mediums 19
photography, art mediums 19
physical, social, emotional or cognite
        challenges 5
physical activity, four types 32
planting seeds 85
political views 21
Post Traumatic Stress Disorder
        (PTSD) 36, 39–41
power 72
Pranayama breaths 36
printmaking, art mediums 19–20
professional relationships 26

race 5–6, 21, 29
rage 100
Regev, D. 14
Registered Art Therapist (ATR) 2
relapse 90–92
relationships *See also* externalizing
religion 5–6, 21, 29
resistance, bypassing 46
response art 95–103
ritual 51–52
Robbins, Arthur 10

safe space 70
safety 72
safety tools: creative mindfulness
        mantra cards 64–66; mandalas
        66–68; safe space 70; tool
        box 68–69
Schmanke, L. 46
sculpture, art mediums 20
second-order representations 12–13
self-esteem 19
self-loathing 32
self portraits 46
self reflection: beggar bowl 74–75; I
        come from 72–74; inside/
        outside box 75; I statements
        75–77; this is me, I am 71; tree
        77–78; what I know for sure
        74–75 *See also* externalizing
self-talk 50–51
sexuality 21
sexual orientation 5
shared history 26
shared history (negative type) 27

shared injury 21
Shore, Annette 3, 5, 13
Siegel, D.J. 12
sleep disorders 35
Snir, S. 14
social anxiety 19, 45, 66, 69
social wellness 26–28
socioeconomic status 21, 25
spiritual wellness 28–29
spontaneous art expression 23
Springham, N. 3, 12
Stonehenge 67
strangers 26
strengths 52
stress disorders 35
struggle container 81–83
Supplemental Nutrition Assistance
        Program (SNAP) 32
Survivor Summit 11

Ter Maat, M.B. 21
this is me, I am 71
tool box 68–69
transitional object 11

trauma 45, 48, 50–51, 79, 81–82,
        85–86, 92
treatment planner 13
tree 77–78
Trump, Donald 29
trust 72
The *12 Steps*, supporting 52–54
The 12 Steps of Alcoholics
        Anonymous 45

unconscious, the 23–24

vicarious trauma 94–103

what does _____ look like? 79–80
what I know for sure 74–75
working with it 85–93; Dear_____
        90; I want you to know 92–93;
        my struggle and my
        environment 89–90; my
        struggles and my relationships
        85–89; planting seeds 85;
        relapse 90–92
worry to relaxation 51–52